Praise for the firs̶ ⟨✓⟩ W9-CFA-494
preventing cancer through nutrition.

"A sensible approach to healthy eating based on the conclusions of the latest nutritional research. While being scientifically sound, the book is also a presentation of appetizing and simple foods which will not require weeks of study to learn to prepare."
—*East West Journal*

"[Her] 1981 book was praised by a wide range of scientists. Now nutritionist Patricia Hausman offers more practical advice."   —*People*

"A responsible, easy-to-follow program for improving nutritional habits in accordance with the National Academy of Sciences report outlining links between diet and cancer. Nutritionist Hausman is a knowledgeable, clear-minded analyst of the nutrition research scene."   —*Kirkus Reviews*

"How specific foods and vitamins can prevent some of the common cancers...distillations of the major research in many cancer-causing and cancer-related areas...how these tips can be translated into use in the daily diet."   —*Publishers Weekly*

"[Among] the top of the heap.... There is a lot of good common sense here, and Hausman isn't selling any panaceas."   —*The Washington Post*

"For the first time, both the National Cancer Institute and the American Cancer Society have published nutritional guidelines aimed at reducing one's chances of getting cancer. Additional advice may be found in several new books, the best of which is a sensible, comprehensive volume by Patricia Hausman called *Foods That Fight Cancer.*"
—*The Bergen Record*, N.J.

—more—

"An accurate, timely presentation of a very important development in the field of cancer prevention. However you do it, buy or borrow, try to read this important book."   —*The Newtown Bee,* Conn.

"Diet can play a role in preventing cancer, the latest research shows...*Foods That Fight Cancer* describes how."   —*USA Today*

ATTENTION: SCHOOLS AND CORPORATIONS

WARNER books are available at quantity discounts with bulk purchase for educational, business, or sales promotional use. For information, please write to: SPECIAL SALES DEPARTMENT, WARNER BOOKS, 666 FIFTH AVENUE, NEW YORK, N Y 10103

**ARE THERE WARNER BOOKS
YOU WANT BUT CANNOT FIND IN YOUR LOCAL STORES?**

You can get any WARNER BOOKS title in print. Simply send title and retail price, plus 50¢ per order and 50¢ per copy to cover mailing and handling costs for each book desired. New York State and California residents add applicable sales tax. Enclose check or money order only, no cash please, to: WARNER BOOKS, PO BOX 690, NEW YORK, N Y 10019

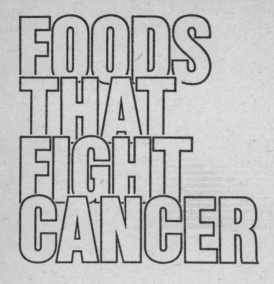

FOODS THAT FIGHT CANCER

A Diet and Vitamin
Program that
Protects the
Entire Family

by Patricia Hausman

WARNER BOOKS

A Warner Communications Company

WARNER BOOKS EDITION

Copyright © 1983 by Patricia Hausman
All rights reserved.

This Warner Books Edition is published by
arrangement with Rawson Associates, 597
Fifth Avenue, New York, N.Y. 10017

Warner Books, Inc.
666 Fifth Avenue
New York, N.Y. 10103

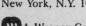A Warner Communications Company

Printed in the United States of America

First Warner Books Printing: May, 1985

10 9 8 7 6 5 4 3 2 1

To my sister, Arlene

A Note to the Reader

This book is based on mounting scientific research linking certain foods to reduced risk of cancer. On the basis of research now available, the author, along with other health professionals, believes that following the recommendations in the book will reduce most people's risk of developing certain forms of cancer. There is no assurance, however, that following these recommendations will prevent cancer in any individual.

Since some people will not tolerate a diet that would be helpful for most, the author urges the reader to consult a physician before making a major change in diet. Of course, anyone who has been diagnosed as suffering from cancer or any other condition should follow the treatment prescribed by a physician. The recommendations in this book are intended as preventive measures, not as a treatment for cancer patients.

Contents

Different Types of Fat...Saturated or Unsaturated?...Fat and Calories...Can Eating Less Fat Be Harmful?

The Recommendation and How to Meet It...An Important Definition...Some Alternatives... Rating the Drinks...A Success Story: Nitrosamines in Beer...A Closer Look at Beer...The Word on Table Wines...Dessert Wines Differ ...The Cocktail Connection...Vodka, Gin, and Rum...Specialty Liquors...The Heart's Desire?...Remember the Calories

Nitrite: Still a Prime Suspect...Meeting the Recommendation...There Are Alternatives!... Healthier Sandwiches...Spice Tips..."Take with Vitamin C"...Rating the Salt-Cured Foods... The Rainbow of Artificial Colors...Which Foods Have Artificial Colors?...The Sweeteners Story ...An Intensive Study of Food Additive Safety ...Each Additive Was Rated...Some Additives Are Nature's Own...Natural Additives with Exotic Names...Some Anti-Cancer Additives... More 100 Percent Natural Additives...Artificial but Safe...The "Uncertain" List...Unsafe as Now Used

Possible Hazards in Food...What's in the Coffee Cup?...About the Different Types of Coffee ...Memo to Tea-Drinkers...Caffeine: A Closeup...The Tannins in Tea...Natural Nitrites and Nitrates...The Mushroom Family...The

List of Tables

Acknowledgments

A hug and kiss to:

* Eleanor Rawson and Toni Sciarra for the best in editorial assistance;
* Susan Cohen and Richard Curtis for their unflagging effort, support, and advice at every step of the way;
* Nutrition Support Headquarters of Minneapolis for the nutritional analysis of the recipes;
* Glen Marcus for an endless supply of ideas, encouragement, and technical advice;
* my friends and family for their understanding and support.

Patricia Hausman
Silver Spring, Maryland
April 1983

1

Good News at Last!

The science of nutrition has come of age. We now know that good nutrition safeguards our health in ways we never dreamed were possible.

A few years ago, I would not have told you that good nutrition would help protect you from cancer. My fellow nutritionists would have laughed at me. My professors at the University of Maryland would have wished that they had never granted me a master's degree in nutrition.

But today, I can tell you that, in my opinion, some simple changes in your diet may very well reduce your chances of developing some forms of cancer. I can show you the scientific research to back my claims. And I doubt that my professors are laughing. They are probably as fascinated as I am by the findings that I am going to tell you about in this book.

A Major Change in Outlook

Most nutritionists will admit that their ideas about diet and health have changed dramatically during the past ten years. I know that mine have. Twelve years ago, when I first began studying nutrition, I revered animal foods, with their high levels of protein, vitamins, and minerals. I didn't have anything against fruits and vegetables, but I was not especially impressed with them. Animal foods, after all, were richer in nutrients.

In 1975, when I became editor of *Nutrition Action* at the Center for Science in the Public Interest, my main concerns were food additives, sugar, and refined grains. At that time, if I heard the words "nutrition" and "cancer" in the same sentence, I would have thought of food additives.

My bible in those days was the *Recommended Dietary Allowances*. It is a book that discusses common nutrients and gives recommended levels of them. These levels, if eaten daily, should meet the needs of most people.

But as I continued to read the latest findings in my field, my opinions started to change.

The first major change in my thinking related to the fat in our diet. It was clear to me that fat was a far bigger problem than sugar or food additives. I saw overwhelming evidence that saturated fats and cholesterol help to cause heart disease.

I also became convinced that salt was a bigger problem than sugar and food additives. It is obvious that salt contributes to high blood pressure. And high blood pressure greatly increases the chances of heart disease.

The Recommended Dietary Allowances Miss the Boat

In 1978, the congressional Subcommittee on Domestic and International Scientific Planning, Analysis and Cooperation asked me to testify at a hearing on the adequacy of the Recommended Dietary Allowances (RDA). At the hearing, I criticized the RDA for neglecting the problems of excessive fat and salt in the diet. I insisted that the RDAs are outdated.

Worse still, I explained, the RDAs can be misleading. The RDA approach to nutrition rewards foods rich in protein, vitamins, and minerals, without any thought about their fat or salt content. As a result, high-fat and high-salt foods that cause our most serious health problems often appear to be the best foods for our health because they have lots of protein and other nutrients.

My concerns about fat were the subject of my first book, *Jack Sprat's Legacy: The Science and Politics of Fat and Cholesterol.*

Fat was also the subject of my first writings on nutrition and cancer. In 1980, I presented a review of more than fifty studies on this subject to the Committee on Diet, Nutrition, and Cancer of the National Academy of Sciences. (I will be telling you all about the committee's conclusions throughout this book.) I was convinced that lowering fat intake would reduce our nation's high rates of breast and colon cancer. But fat was the only aspect of our diet that I felt played a role in causing cancer.

On each of these occasions, I received letters and phone calls from people who could not believe that it was the same Patricia Hausman talking. But none of them could convince me to go back to my earlier beliefs. I realized just how much my convictions had changed.

Many Aspects of Diet Can Help Prevent Cancer

Today, I look back at that testimony about the RDAs, my paper on fat and cancer, and my first book, and say that these writings, too, are outdated.

Fat and salt are still serious problems. But only recently did I realize that there are new issues in nutrition that are just as important as eating less fat and salt.

These new issues pertain to nutrition and cancer. And for a pleasant change, the most important of these new issues relate to substances in food that can protect against cancer. I, too, was growing weary of all the warnings about the latest cancer-causing chemical in food. But relief is in sight. Instead of hearing only negatives, *we will be hearing more about findings that link certain foods to prevention of cancer.*

Already there are good research studies showing that some foods have anti-cancer potential. Stay tuned and I will tell you about them.

The Bright Future Ahead

It has been more than four decades since Congress passed the National Cancer Institute Act. That act created the National Cancer Institute and made cancer a major topic of medical research.

For many years, the war against cancer was a frustrating one; the hoped-for breakthrough that would do for cancer what penicillin did for infections seemed ever further away.

Finally, there is reason for hope. "Most common cancers are potentially preventable," concluded the blue-ribbon Committee on Diet, Nutrition and Cancer of the National Academy of Sciences in June of 1982. The committee went on to say that most common forms of cancer "appear to be determined more by habit, diet, and custom than by genetic differences."

The committee declined to say precisely how much cancer can be prevented by changes in diet. But in a report prepared for Congress's Office of Technology Assessment, two well-known cancer experts made some rough estimates. They ventured that changes in diet *might reduce U.S. cancer rates by 35 percent.*

This book will help you design a diet for yourself that allows you to take advantage of the research that led to these scientists' conclusions.

Diet May Help Prevent Ten Forms of Cancer

There are many different kinds of cancer, of course. I, as well as many of my colleagues, believe that good nutrition can help to prevent many though not all of them. In this book, we'll be talking about the things that you can do to protect yourself from those cancers that are sensitive to diet.

The Committee on Diet, Nutrition, and Cancer cited the following cancers as among those that may be prevented by good nutrition:

- breast cancer—the form of cancer most common among American women
- colon cancer—a form that is very common in both sexes
- lung cancer—the most common type of cancer in American men

The Committee also found evidence that diet may also help prevent at least seven other forms of cancer: cancers of the mouth and throat, esophagus, stomach, prostate, ovary, uterus, and rectum.

Help for Smokers and Gourmets

I would like to point out to you a very positive aspect of the relationship between nutrition and cancer. Most of us have found it difficult—if not impossible—to do what is best for our health at all times. Thousands of people, for instance, have tried to stop smoking—without success. They are probably tired of hearing only the "stop smoking" message.

Of course, those who urge smokers to stop are absolutely right. There is no better way to prevent lung cancer than to kick the habit. But research now shows that smokers who eat diets rich in vitamin A are less likely to have lung cancer than smokers who do not. In other words, a diet high in vitamin A seems to be helping those who cannot seem to part with their cigarettes.

Don't get me wrong. I am not telling you that eating lots of fruits and vegetables makes smoking okay. But the evidence is good that it helps protect smokers to some degree.

Since I am known mostly for my work on fat and cholesterol, I often hear people complain that high-fat foods taste too good to pass up. (Actually, I advocate eating *less* fat, not none at all.) But I know health-minded people who are also gourmet cooks. Parting with high-fat foods is sometimes more than they are willing to do.

Again, I will not tell you that a high-fiber diet can do away with all the risks posed by a diet rich in fat. But there is evidence that fiber does counteract the ill effects of fat to some degree. For the most part, colon cancer is the issue here. Fat promotes this form of cancer. But I think that certain high-fiber foods can undo some of the damage. In the chapter on fiber, I will tell you why.

Cured meats are another popular food that some people cannot bear to give up. In college, I had a roommate who insisted that she could not live without bacon. She knew all about the reports that cooked bacon often contained trouble-makers called nitrosamines. Tiny amounts of nitrosamines cause cancer in a long list of animals.

Along comes research showing that vitamin C can help prevent nitrosamines from forming. In some instances, vitamin C has completely blocked the reaction that produces nitrosamines; in other cases, it reduces the amount that forms. If you have noticed vitamin C (sometimes listed as ascorbate) on the label of your bacon packages lately, this is one reason why.

In short, new findings in nutrition and cancer have shown ways that good nutrition can counteract our weaknesses. There is every reason to be excited by these findings—as long as we keep in mind that nutrition cannot eliminate all risks. But it can reduce their impact.

There is another happy aspect to the story of nutrition and cancer. It is now obvious that the same diet that can reduce your risk of cancer will also give you added protection from other health problems. Heart disease, diabetes, diverticulosis—even obesity— are among the conditions that can benefit from the same diet that you will learn about in this book.

Tailoring a Diet to Your Special Needs

How can a book give advice on preventing cancer when each of us has different genes? When some work with hazardous chemicals and others do not?

When some smoke cigarettes, while others avoid even a room with smokers in it?

I have tried to cope with what might be called our individuality. Each chapter begins with a prominent notice listing conditions that call for special attention to the food element discussed in that chapter. The purpose of this introductory note is to help you to identify the dietary changes that can best protect you. For example:

- Those with a family history of breast, ovary, or prostate cancer will want to pay special attention to the chapter about fat.
- Men and women who work with hazardous chemicals should carefully read the sections on vitamins A and C.
- Smokers will want to emphasize the chapters about vitamin A and alcohol.

Nonetheless, this book is not intended as a substitute for your doctor. If you have a condition that puts you at extra risk of cancer, you should discuss your diet with your doctor. Chances are good that you can take measures to help reduce that extra risk.

It Is Not Too Late

People often say to me, "I have been eating this way my entire life. There is nothing to be gained by changing at this point in my life."

They seem to think the damage has been irreversibly done, and one's only course of action is to await the inevitable bad news. It is a shame that some people feel this way, not only because hopelessness is a sorry state, but also because there is good scientific evidence that even late-life changes can influence the course of some forms of cancer, as well as heart disease.

During the years that I studied heart disease, I was often amazed that men who switched to cholesterol-lowering diets during their forties, fifties, and even sixties experienced some benefit to their heart health. I was frankly surprised when three solemn-looking, official-sounding heart experts held a press conference at the American Heart Association's annual meeting and announced that hardening of the arteries can be reversed under some conditions.

Later, when I studied nutrition and colon cancer, I found that even late-life changes affect the course of the disease. Studies of Japanese immigrants have found that Japanese men who came to the United States during middle age did not retain the low risk of colon cancer found in their native land. On the contrary, they quickly experienced almost the same high rates of colon cancer as American men.

It might be a fluke, I thought, one of those things that shows up in one study, never to be found again. But not so. Similar studies found that Polish immigrants, too, no longer experienced the low colon cancer rates found in their native land. Not long after they came to the United States, their colon cancer rates started to resemble those of the U.S. population. Norwegian immigrants, too, soon found themselves with colon cancer rates that more closely resembled the rate found in the United States than in Norway.

Scientists have a good idea of what happened. On moving to the United States, Japanese men increased their fat intake. Had they continued to eat the traditional, low-fat Japanese diet, they probably would have prevented many cases of colon cancer. An increase in fat intake might also account for high colon cancer rates among immigrants from other countries too.

Though we may never be able to account for every extra case of colon cancer among these adult immigrants, we can draw some conclusions from this research. These findings tell us that the chance of developing colon cancer can be influenced late in life.

What's Happening in Later Life

These findings fit current thinking among cancer scientists. They now believe that cancer has several stages. In the early stage, a cell in the body is damaged. Whether it grows into cancer depends on a series of other stages.

One of the later stages is called promotion. During this phase, factors such as nutrition can act to keep the cancer growing. They can also fight the cancer and slow—or stop—its growth.

The stories of Japanese, Polish, and Norwegian migrants tell us that changes in the promotional stage—one of the last stages of colon cancer—can influence whether the disease develops.

We can hope that future research will show whether nutrition can affect cancer once it is diagnosed. Years ago, a team of scientists reported that breast cancer patients in Japan fared significantly better than American women with breast cancer. Can the lower-fat Japanese diet explain this result? It certainly is worthy of testing.

Of course, for maximum benefit, cancer-preventing food habits should be developed early in life. We have every reason to believe that the earlier such measures are adopted, the better the outcome will be.

For Our Children's Sake

In June of 1982, the Committee on Diet, Nutrition, and Cancer of the National Academy of Sciences released its first report on nutrition and cancer prevention. In the upcoming chapters, we will be looking at each of the committee's recommendations in detail.

One notable aspect of the committee's recommendations pertains to children. The group expressed its belief that children as well as adults should be following its recommendations.

"The dietary pattern we suggest should be implemented at the time children start participating in the family meals," explained Dr. Walter Mertz, a member of the committee. The committee recommended that we eat less fat. Diets lower in fat would benefit most of us, but children under one year of age should not be given low-fat diets. Infants grow rapidly during their first year of life. A diet low in fat may not provide enough calories for their needs.

Childhood Can Be Most Important

There are several reasons why cancer scientists believe that children, too, should eat diets designed to prevent cancer. First, as we all know, habits are not easy to break. If we learned sound food habits early in life, as adults we probably would find it easier to choose the foods best for our health.

And of course it makes sense that the longer a

recommendation is followed, the better the benefit will be.

There is a third reason to emphasize cancer-preventing food habits in childhood. Some cancers seem to be influenced most strongly by childhood and/or adolescence.

Studies of migrating populations support this idea. Japanese women who came to the United States as adults retained the low risk of breast cancer seen in their homeland. But the children of these women born in the United States do not have the same low rates.

Other studies support this concept. Women exposed to radiation as adults are less likely to have breast cancer than those exposed during their teen years. And women who bear children early in life have less risk than those who have their first child late in life. It is obvious that for this form of cancer, lifestyle during our first twenty or thirty years of life is particularly important.

There is reason to believe that some other forms of cancer are particularly influenced by the practices of early life. Cancers of the stomach and prostate gland also seem most sensitive to our early-life habits.

Again, the health records of our nation's immigrants tell the tale. Japanese migrants who came to the United States as adults still suffered the high stomach cancer rates found in their native land. As consolation, though, these Japanese men retained the extremely low rate of prostate cancer found in Japan.

For immigrants from six European countries, the story was the same. Their stomach cancer rates were closer to the rate of their native land—not the rate of their new country.

These findings tell us that early-life factors probably count most when it comes to these two forms of cancer.

All things considered, then, both young and old can gain from food habits that reduce the risk of cancer.

Good Health and *Good Eating*

You might not believe me, but most nutritionists do love to eat. In fact, I am willing to bet that most of us think about food more than the average person does. Put me in that category. I love to cook and read about food. Above all, I love to eat!

When I first considered writing books about nutrition, I decided I would not do it unless I could convince myself that my recommendations could please both the palate and the body. I am happy to say that I have convinced myself about a hundred times—at least.

During the past few years, I have spent thousands of hours in the kitchen experimenting. I have had my share of failures and flops, but also some spectacular successes. I have my own ways of making low-fat, low-salt, highly nutritious food taste good. Throughout the book, you'll learn about them.

I will also be telling you about kitchenware that helps make good nutrition taste very good. Ordering information, of course, is included.

I have designed some recipes that combine foods high in vitamin C with those that contain sodium nitrite. These recipes are for people who cannot resist cured foods but also want to take sensible precautions for their health.

Nutrition Information That
Anyone Can Understand

Each recipe in the book is followed by important nutrition information. This will allow you to choose those recipes that best meet your own special needs.

Rather than present long lists of numbers, I have translated these nutrient values into a simple rating system. A quick glance at the nutrient rating will help you identify the recipes that are lowest in fat, highest in vitamin A and C, or suitable for a number of special diets. The numbers behind the ratings are explained in the beginning of the recipe section.

If vitamin A is your top priority, look for recipes with three stars for vitamin A. Ditto for fiber and vitamin C.

If you have to watch your fat or sodium, favor the recipes that rate three stars for these two items. Such recipes have low levels of these troublemakers.

I have presented some of my very favorite recipes in this book. I do hope you'll try them.

2

The Case for Prevention

"The time to redirect our research efforts and to apply the results to prevention [of cancer] is NOW."

With these words, Dr. John Weisburger urged his fellow scientists to put more effort into preventing cancer. Weisburger is vice-president of the American Health Foundation, a New York organization dedicated to preventive medicine. As he knows, most of our cancer research dollars have been spent on treatment. Prevention has been all but forgotten.

Most cancer scientists are well aware that gains have been made in cancer treatment. To name a few:

- Treatment of leukemia has improved dramatically in the past decade. Survival rates have more than doubled for some forms of the disease.
- During 1970 to 1973, white males with cancers of the colon, rectum, and bladder were more likely to survive for five or more years than patients who had these diseases between 1960 and 1963.
- Black men with cancers of the stomach, prostate gland, and bladder showed better survival rates during the 1970s than during the 1960s.
- During the last decade, both white and black women scored significant gains against cancers of the breast, colon, rectum, uterus, and cervix.

More Progress Is Possible

Why are cancer scientists stressing prevention of cancer when treatment is getting better and better?

The answer is simple. At this time, we don't have a cure for any form of cancer that works 100 percent of the time. Good treatments exist for some but not all forms of the disease. Doctors can't promise a cure to any cancer patient.

Who wouldn't prefer preventing the disease to facing the uncertain outcome of our current treatments—even if the chances for recovery are good?

Who wouldn't prefer prevention to missing time from work and favorite activities for treatment?

And who wouldn't prefer prevention to worrying about the effects of cancer on our friends and family? Like all diseases, cancer has its direct costs in treatment and lost work time. But the emotional costs can't be measured.

Preventive efforts could spare us from these costs. No one knows how many cases of cancer will be eliminated by preventive medicine. But scientists have estimated that anywhere from 30 to 60 percent of Americans who eventually develop cancer might be spared by good nutrition.

Prevention Is Now a Priority

It is not easy to convince scientists to change their outlook. Once a way of thinking takes hold, it often can't be changed for decades.

Four decades ago, every scientist and doctor in the world was inspired by the success story of penicillin. Almost overnight, there was a powerful weapon that could do away with life-threatening diseases. No wonder that researchers set out to find a drug that would also wipe out cancer.

But while the search was on, bits and pieces of information about the origins of cancer were accumulating. Eventually, the bits and pieces became a mountain. The mountain of evidence *has convinced me, as well as the Committee on Diet, Nutrition, and Cancer, that most forms of cancer can be prevented.*

This evidence has started a revolution among cancer scientists. The very people who have spent their lifetimes looking for a cancer cure are now urging us to do more to prevent cancer.

Overwhelming Evidence for Prevention

What changed their minds? It wasn't any one study, but rather a long list of them. For example:

- Rates of colon and breast cancer vary dramatically throughout the world. Some nations, such as Japan, Thailand, and the Philippines, have only one-fifth as much breast cancer as many Western nations. The United States, Denmark, and the Netherlands have five times the breast cancer rate of these low-risk countries.
- Within a country, cancers of the colon and breast are often more common among the rich than the poor. Stomach cancer is often more common among the poor.
- Immigrants often leave behind the forms of cancer that were common in their native land. If they do develop cancer, it usually is one that is common in their new country.

The meaning of these findings is clear. If some countries can manage to have low rates of breast cancer, it is obvious that the disease does not have to be common. There is every reason to believe that it can (and should) be a rare disease.

If the rich can avoid some forms of cancer, so can the poor. All that we have to do is find out what the secrets of prevention are—and make sure that everyone has access to them.

The wealthy can benefit, too, by adopting the habits that protect poor people from breast and colon cancers. If the poor can escape these forms of cancer, there is no reason why the wealthy cannot.

And if migrating from one country can cut the chances of developing various forms of cancer, it is clear that cancer is not written onto our genes. If it were, Japanese-Americans would have the high rates of stomach cancer of the Japanese mainland. Instead, they have the very low rates found among the general U.S. population.

Faced with these facts, who can possibly believe that cancer is an unavoidable part of life? Anyone who tells you that "life is carcinogenic" is simply a pessimist, and an unscientific one at that.

The Food Habits That Help

As I said earlier, the Committee on Diet, Nutrition, and Cancer concluded that good nutrition may help prevent many—but not all—forms of cancer. Good nutrition refers to a half dozen practices that are strongly linked to reduced rates of cancer. For instance:

• Diets rich in vitamin A are linked to reduced rates of cancers of the lung, bladder, esophagus, and throat.

- People who eat generous amounts of foods rich in vitamin C have below average rates of stomach and esophageal cancer.
- Foods in the cabbage family appear to contain substances that block the action of cancer-causing chemicals.
- Diets rich in some forms of fiber go hand in hand with lower rates of colon cancer.
- Stomach cancer is less common where diets contain few highly pickled or cured foods.
- Cancers of the breast, colon, prostate gland, and uterus are rare where diets are low in fat.
- Nutrient deficiencies and consumption of moldy foods are linked to liver cancer.

Diet May Prevent Our Most Common Cancers

It is no wonder that this is important news. Some of the most common cancers in the United States are the very ones that good nutrition can help to prevent.

In fact, nutrition shows promise in preventing the four most common forms of cancer among American men and women. For men, these are cancers of the lung, prostate gland, colon and rectum, and bladder. For women, breast cancer is first, followed by cancers of the colon and rectum, uterus, and lung.

There is evidence that good nutrition may help prevent some forms of cancer in addition to the ones mentioned above. I will tell you about such links in the upcoming chapters. I tell about these links only for your information, however, and not with any recommendation that you act as yet. It is best to concentrate only on those dietary habits that are strongly linked to lower rates of cancer.

For the record, I would also like to mention the forms of cancer that have not been linked to diet. Cancers of the brain, eye, and thyroid gland show no relationship to diet, nor do leukemia and Hodgkin's disease. Fortunately, none of these are on the list of the most common cancers in the United States.

Voices for Prevention

George Gallup should take a few polls among scientists and not just among registered voters. We often hear that a notion is controversial among scientists, but rarely does anyone stop to measure just how controversial the idea truly is.

The notion that good nutrition can reduce the chance of developing cancer may be new, but it is not a hotly debated idea. On the contrary, many knowledgeable scientists now favor dietary practices designed to protect us from cancer.

The most important dietary advice has come from the group known as the Committee on Diet, Nutrition, and Cancer.

In 1980, the federal government's National Cancer Institute asked the National Academy of Sciences to review everything that is known about nutrition and cancer. The academy agreed and set up the Committee on Diet, Nutrition, and Cancer to conduct the study. The committee was a group of highly respected scientists from universities and government agencies.

It took the committee scientists two years to complete their study. In June of 1982, the panel presented its conclusions.

"Our most general conclusion is that the evidence is increasingly impressive that what we eat does affect our chances of getting cancer, especially particular kinds of cancer," explained Dr. Clifford Grobstein, chairman of the committee.

"This is, believe it or not, good news," he continued. "It means that by controlling what we eat we may prevent diet-sensitive cancers—possibly an easier task than eradicating them after they have taken hold. An ounce of prevention . . . may be on the horizon."

The Official Anti-Cancer Advice

As that "ounce of prevention," Dr. Grobstein and his committee offered these words of advice:

- Eat fruits, vegetables, and whole grain cereal products daily—especially those fruits and vegetables rich in vitamins A and C. Also emphasize those vegetables belonging to the cabbage family.
- Reduce fat intake by 25 percent.
- Eat very little salt-cured, salt-pickled, and smoked foods, such as sausages, ham, bacon, bologna, and hot dogs.
- Drink alcohol only in moderation.

More Support for Preventive Action

The recommendations of the Committee on Diet, Nutrition, and Cancer are the most authoritative advice on the subject of nutrition and cancer. In editorials, both the *New York Times* and the *Washington Post* urged us to follow the Committee's advice.

"Since absolutely conclusive evidence will take years to develop, the Committee members felt that the evidence justifies action now," wrote the *Washington Post*. "Surely they are right."

But it is not just the press that agrees with the

Committee on Diet, Nutrition, and Cancer. In 1979, for instance, the National Cancer Institute (a part of the National Institutes of Health) issued its own diet advice to the public.

Like the Committee on Diet, Nutrition, and Cancer, the National Cancer Institute recommended eating ample amounts of fruits and vegetables. The institute also advised cutting back on fat, drinking only moderate amounts of alcohol, and choosing more fiber-containing foods. Obesity and high-dose vitamin supplements should be avoided, said the institute.

It All Began in the Senate

Odd as it may seem, however, the first statement on nutrition and cancer was not issued by scientists. On the contrary, it was released by politicians.

In 1977, the Senate select committee on Nutrition and Human Needs issued a report that made history. Called *Dietary Goals for the United States*, the report was the first to suggest food habits that can prevent cancer. It recommended eating more fruits, vegetables, and whole grains—and less fat.

The *Dietary Goals* report won the attention of scientists throughout the country and the world. George McGovern, who was then chairman of the Senate Select Committee, said that he never imagined that the report would draw as much attention as it did.

But it was a good—if not great—thing that so many noticed the report. Five years after its publication, McGovern's *Dietary Goals* report has become the official advice of our most knowledgeable cancer experts. Nothing in the 1982 report of the Committee on Diet, Nutrition, and Cancer contradicts the advice in *Dietary Goals for the United States*.

Adding the Latest Findings

The report of the Committee on Diet, Nutrition, and Cancer, though, includes findings that were not available when the *Dietary Goals for the United States* was in process. In a sense, the report of the Committee on Diet, Nutrition, and Cancer is an updated version of the *Dietary Goals*.

The rest of this book will be devoted to the report by the Committee on Diet, Nutrition, and Cancer because this report has the very latest in research findings. I have included a chapter on each important area of the committee's report.

The remaining chapters of this book have a similar format. First, we will look at the forms of cancer that each food element can prevent. The committee's recommendation for that food substance will follow.

After describing the recommendation, I will give you the nutrition information that you need to meet the committee's advice. I will be telling you not just about the foods that enable you to meet the recommendation but also about how to prepare them. I'll give some ideas for planning menus around the appropriate foods. And you'll also find money-saving information in many chapters.

For the skeptic, each chapter includes a discussion of both the pluses and minuses of the food element in question. And for the optimist, we will look at other benefits to be reaped from following the committee's advice.

The committee's recommendations are remarkably similar to expert advice for preventing other common diseases. Let's start, now, to look at each recommendation in detail.

3

Vitamin A

Focus on this chapter if you smoke cigarettes, work with hazardous chemicals, or eat pickled or cured foods often. If your doctor has told you that you have a premalignant condition of the esophagus, ask for personalized dietary advice on a regular basis.

From all over the world have come the most exciting findings ever reported about vitamin A. More than a dozen studies have linked diets rich in vitamin A to a surprising amount of protection against some forms of cancer.

In Chicago, scientists found only two cases of lung cancer among five hundred men, including some smokers, who ate many fruits and vegetables rich in vitamin A. That was only one-seventh as many lung cancer cases as were found in 500 men who ate few of these foods.

And in Norway, the findings were no different. Men who ate many vegetables rich in vitamin A had only one-third as much lung cancer as those eating little of these foods.

In Japan, the story was the same. Researchers found 30 percent fewer cases of lung cancer among people who ate vegetables rich in vitamin A every day. The daily vegetable eaters also had lower rates of stomach cancer.

Cancer scientists have been so fascinated by these findings that the ability of vitamin A to protect us from cancer has become one of their top interests. Many are already convinced that we should be eating more foods rich in vitamin A. The Committee on Diet, Nutrition, and Cancer of the National Academy of Sciences has urged us to do so.

Studies have linked a diet rich in vitamin A to protection from cancer in eight different organs. The evidence is strongest for cancer of the lung, stomach, or esophagus.

But there is more good news. Research also ties vitamin A to protection from cancers of the mouth, colon, rectum, prostate, and bladder. There is less evidence here than for lung, stomach, and esophageal cancer. But there is enough to merit our attention.

Three Types of Vitamin A

"Vitamin A" is a very general term. It refers to several substances that can take care of the body's need for this nutrient.

For many of the body's functions that need vitamin A, any form will do. But in cancer prevention, the picture looks different. As things stand right now, *it seems that only some kinds of vitamin A may protect against cancer.*

For this reason, it is important to be aware of the three kinds of vitamin A in food.

- Retinol is the vitamin A in animal foods.
- Carotene (or beta-carotene) is the main kind of vitamin A in fruits and vegetables.

- Carotenoids are other forms of vitamin A found in fruits and vegetables. They are a very minor source of vitamin A.

Of these different kinds of vitamin A, carotene is linked most strongly to protection from cancer.

Vitamin A Supplements Are Different

Of course, we can also get vitamin A from pills. The form used in vitamin compounds is not carotene or retinol. It usually is a synthetic form of vitamin A called vitamin A palmitate. Little research has been done on the ability of this kind of vitamin A to protect against cancer.

For this reason, it is not a good idea to rely on vitamin A pills to reduce your risk of cancer. Scientists simply don't know if this type of vitamin A has any value in preventing cancer.

You may also be aware that the kind of vitamin A usually contained in vitamin capsules or tablets can be toxic if taken in very high doses. In a later section, we will look at this possibility in greater detail.

Newspapers and magazines have published some articles about special forms of vitamin A that show remarkable anti-cancer potential in laboratory animals. Scientists have used these forms of vitamin A, called retinoids, to block cancers of the lung, bladder, and breast in test animals.

Retinoids may be on the drugstore shelves someday. But right now they are not for sale. Their use is strictly experimental.

The Recommendation and How to Meet It

The Committee on Diet, Nutrition, and Cancer recommends daily consumption of fruits and vegetables. The committee advises us to emphasize those fruits and vegetables that are rich in carotene, the most important kind of vitamin A in plant foods.

To help in selecting foods, the Committee prepared the following chart which classifies foods as low, medium, or high in carotene.

Carotene in Fruits and Vegetables		
Low*	Medium**	High***
Apples	Brussels sprouts	Apricots
Bananas	Corn (yellow)	Asparagus
Cabbage	Green beans	Broccoli
Cauliflower	Green pepper	Cantaloupe
Celery	Peas	Carrots
Cherries	Summer squash	Dark green leafy
Cucumbers	Watermelon	vegetables
Grapes		Kale
Grapefruit		Mangoes
Iceberg lettuce		Peaches
Kohlrabi		Pumpkins
Lemons		Romaine lettuce
Limes		Spinach
Oranges		Sweet potatoes
Pears		Tomatoes
Pineapple		Winter squash
Plums		
Potatoes (white)		
Raspberries		
Strawberries		
Tangerines		

continued on p. 28

Carotene in Fruits and Vegetables (continued)

Low*   Medium**   High***

* Low: Less than 500 IU vitamin A per serving.
**Medium: 500 to 1000 IU vitamin A per serving.
*** High: More than 1000 IU vitamin A per serving.
Chart adapted from a 1982 compilation by the Committee on Diet, Nutrition, and Cancer, National Academy of Sciences.

Color Is the Clue

Color is sometimes the key to judging the carotene in fruits and vegetables. Deep green and yellow vegetables are usually very good sources of vitamin A. But lighter versions of the same foods are not. For example:

- Green asparagus is rich in vitamin A. The bleached white asparagus has only one-tenth as much!
- Romaine lettuce provides four times as much vitamin A as iceberg lettuce.
- Yellow corn has more vitamin A than white corn.
- Green beans have more vitamin A than wax beans.

Here is my favorite piece of vitamin A trivia: frozen chopped broccoli has one-third more vitamin A than the frozen spears. I am willing to bet that the leaves in the chopped version make the difference. Their deep green color is a sure sign of vitamin A!

Though fruits and vegetables supply almost half of our vitamin A, other foods do have significant amounts. Meat, poultry, and fish provide about one-fourth of the vitamin A in the American diet; dairy products give another 15 percent or so. Eggs and other foods supply a little less than 10 percent.

But it is not known whether the vitamin A in most animal foods has any value in cancer prevention. That is why the Committee on Diet, Nutrition, and Cancer restricted its recommendations to fruits and vegetables.

How Much Is Enough?

The Committee on Diet, Nutrition, and Cancer did not tell us exactly how much vitamin A to eat each day. But I will try to give some rough guidelines.

For decades, nutritionists have recommended that we eat four or more servings of fruits and vegetables each day. It is a good idea to ensure that at least two to three of these servings are rich in vitamin A. I try to eat a fruit or vegetable rich in vitamin A at every meal.

I have been following my own advice for quite a while. So I can tell you that eventually you find yourself eating fruits and vegetables rich in vitamin A almost automatically.

It's Easy to Do

Here are a few simple ways to get your vitamin A intake where the experts think it should be:

- Eat a salad every day, using lettuce that is dark green (such as romaine) and other carotene-rich ingredients such as tomatoes, green pepper, and carrots.
- Drink juices daily that are high in vitamin A,

such as apricot nectar, tomato juice, or vegetable juice cocktail.

- Substitute sweet potatoes for white potatoes.
- Keep a jar of dried apricots handy in the kitchen or on the table. If you can nibble during the day without gaining weight, keep a jar of apricots on your desk or near your work area.
- Top cereal with fruits rich in vitamin A.
- Keep carrot sticks in cold water on hand as a snack.
- Add parsley to recipes—and eat it.
- Use tomato sauce instead of white sauce on pasta and main dishes.
- Add chopped green pepper to chicken and tuna salads.

Of course, there are more exotic approaches, too. How about a high-carotene pizza using broccoli, green beans, and/or green pepper for "extras"? Or learning to cook in a wok. Stir-fried vegetables can be a novelty, and they are healthful if you use only small amounts of oil.

Proclaim one or more nights of the week as "vegetarian night" around your house and see how delicious and healthful eating less meat can be.

Here is another tip: substitute sweet potatoes for white potatoes not just as a vegetable but in some of the many dishes made with potatoes. I used to make potato pancakes and potato scones; now I make sweet potato pancakes and sweet potato biscuits. And sweet potatoes aren't the only vegetable suitable for baking. Pumpkin is another. My pumpkin bread has received especially good reviews. Turn to the recipe section for my recipes.

Making the Most of Our Vitamin A

If you are nutrition-minded, you probably try not to lose nutrients in cooking.

But with vitamin A, you don't have to worry. It is tough stuff; pretty much indifferent to water, heat, and even long periods of storage. Vitamin A does not dissolve in water, so it does not leach into water used in cooking.

Water not only doesn't hurt vitamin A, but probably helps us to make the most of it. Cooking raw vegetables makes some nutrients more accessible to the body. Vitamin A is one of them.

Like vitamins D, E, and K, vitamin A is soluble in fat. This means that your body needs fat to absorb it. Will cutting back on fat leave you without enough to absorb vitamin A? The chances are almost nil.

It is amazing how little fat your body needs to absorb vitamin A. In fact, people who eat only one-fourth as much fat as the typical American show no signs of vitamin A deficiency! So cutting fat down to a moderate level, as recommended by the Committee on Diet, Nutrition, and Cancer, is not going to give you a deficiency of vitamin A. What it will do is make you healthier.

The Bargain-Hunter's Guide

If you are like me, you're concerned not only with the healthfulness of your diet but also its cost.

My first reaction to the vitamin A advice was, "But some of those foods are so expensive!" Fortunately for me, I decided to think twice.

I used to look only at the price tag. Then I

decided to consider the "bang for the buck." What good is a food that costs only ten cents but has little nutrient value?

So I sat down with my grocery bill and my tables of food composition. I computed the cost of getting 1000 international units (IU) of vitamin A from dozens of different foods. An international unit is a standard measure of vitamin A, just as a milligram (mg) is the standard measure for vitamin C.

The results took me by surprise. Suddenly, foods that had always looked expensive became bargains.

Here is one example. In the Washington, D.C., area, where I live, dried apricots sell for four to six dollars a pound—on a par with top cuts of meat. But a handful of dried apricots have so much vitamin A that it costs less to get 1000 IU of this vitamin from apricots than from lots of other foods. At a cost of four dollars a pound, it costs only eight cents to get 1000 IU of vitamin A from dried apricots. Two large dried apricots or three medium ones supply about 1000 IU of the vitamin.

Here are some of the best buys for vitamin A:

- Canned carrots and canned sweet potatoes provide 1000 IU of vitamin A for only a penny!
- Runners-up, at two cents per 1000 IU, are fresh carrots, canned pumpkin, canned or frozen spinach, canned mustard or turnip greens, and fresh kale.
- Cooked frozen squash and fresh spinach, along with frozen collards, mustard or turnip greens come in third, at three cents per 1000 IU.

The chart on pages 33 and 34 shows how much of these foods is needed to provide the 1000 IU.

You may be wondering why I picked the level of 1000 IU. I did so because this is a reasonable amount for a serving of a food to provide. This level of vitamin A equals 20 percent of the RDA for adult men and 25 percent for adult women.

I was so taken with my findings that I made the chart that follows. It shows the cost of getting 1000 international units of vitamin A from various fruits and vegetables. The quantities tell you how much of the food is needed to supply 1000 IU of vitamin A.

My chart showed me that some frozen foods are a better buy than fresh when it comes to vitamin A. So I don't feel guilty that I sometimes use frozen foods for their convenience. I rarely buy canned vegetables, though, even those that are the cheapest sources of vitamin A. Canned vegetables often have far too much salt.

Bang for the Buck
Cost of 1000 IU Vitamin A from Fruits and Vegetables

1¢:	Carrots, canned, ⅓ of a 2″ piece
	Sweet potatoes, canned, 1 piece, 1″ in diameter and length
2¢:	Sweet potatoes, fresh, 1 tablespoon, cooked and mashed
	Carrots, fresh, raw, ⅛ of a 7″ piece
	Spinach, canned or frozen, 1 tablespoon
	Pumpkin, canned, ½ tablespoon
	Kale, mustard greens, or turnip greens, fresh, ⅛ cup
3¢:	Spinach, fresh, ¼ cup, raw
	Collards, frozen, 1½ tablespoons
	Mustard or turnip greens, frozen, ⅛ cup
	Squash, frozen, ⅛ cup
4¢:	Mixed vegetables, frozen, ⅛ cup
6–8¢:	Cantaloupe, fresh, ¼ cup, pieces
	Mango, ⅛ cup, pieces
	Tomato juice, ½ cup
	Broccoli, frozen, ¼ cup
	Apricots, dried, 2 large or 3 medium

continued on page 34

Bang for the Buck (continued)
Cost of 1000 IU Vitamin A from Fruits and Vegetables

12–14¢:   Apricots, canned, 2 halves
          Peaches, fresh, 1 medium or ½ large
          Nectarines, fresh, ½
          Romaine lettuce, 1 cup
          Broccoli, fresh, ¼ cup
15–20¢:   Watermelon, fresh, 1 cup, diced
          Tomatoes, canned, ½ cup
          Acorn squash, fresh, ¼, baked
21–25¢:   Peas, canned, 1 cup
          Tomatoes, fresh, 1
26–30¢:   Peas, frozen, 1 cup
          Peaches, canned, 1 cup
          Papaya, fresh, ½ cup, diced
          Yellow corn, canned, 1⅓ cups
          Yellow summer squash, fresh, 1½ cups, sliced
40–50¢:   Green beans, fresh, 1½ cups
          Green beans, frozen, 1¼ cups
51–60¢:   Brussels sprouts, frozen, 1 cup
          Green beans, canned, 1½ cups
          Yellow corn, frozen, 1¾ cups
          Green pepper, fresh, 3 medium or 1½ large
61–75¢:   Green asparagus, canned, ½ cup
          Green asparagus, fresh, 8 medium spears
          Green asparagus, frozen, ⅔ cup

Costs reflect July 1982 prices in a Washington, D.C., supermarket. Whenever possible, costs for canned items are based on a one-pound can. For frozen items, costs are based on a 10-ounce box.
Values assume that food is cooked unless otherwise noted.

More Benefits of Fruits and Vegetables

I would tell you to eat more fruits and vegetables even if I didn't believe that their carotene has anti-cancer potential, for these foods do much more for you.

With the exception of avocados and coconut, fruits and vegetables are admirably low in fat. The low rates of breast and colon cancer among people who eat low-fat diets tell us that eating more low-fat foods should help protect us from these forms of cancer.

Aside from the unique coconut, fruits and vegetables lack the notorious threesome that fuels heart disease: saturated fat, cholesterol, and sodium. Coconut, however, is high in saturated fat.

Another plus in fruits and vegetables is dietary fiber. There are different kinds of fiber, just as there are different kinds of vitamin A. Fruits and vegetables contain a type of fiber called pectin. When eaten in large amounts, it helps to control blood cholesterol. Six or more servings a day are probably needed for an effect.

Pectin, as well as other kinds of fiber in fruits and vegetables, helps to control the blood sugar level too. This aids diabetics. New diabetic diets often call for six or more servings of fruits and vegetables.

Even those of us who do not have diabetes may benefit from fiber's effect on blood sugar. After a meal low in fiber, the blood sugar can rise sharply, then fall abruptly. Fatigue, hunger, and irritability can set in when this happens. By preventing these sharp ups and downs in the blood sugar, the fiber in fruits and vegetables can help to prevent these symptoms.

We will talk more about fiber in a later chapter.

Are There Hazards?

No doubt about it, too much vitamin A can spell trouble. But it depends on which form of vitamin A you are consuming.

You cannot overdose on the carotene in fruits and vegetables. That is, it cannot make you sick. It can cause a discoloring of the skin, however. If eaten in large amounts, the carotene in fruits and vegetables can be deposited in your skin. The yellowing of the skin is the only symptom. It usually will go away within a few weeks of lowering carotene intake. There is no known harm from this condition.

For most people, the surest way to overdose on vitamin A is to take high-dose vitamin supplements. At very high levels, vitamin A pills can cause a toxic reaction. The classic symptoms are headaches, bone pain, loss of appetite, skin rashes, fatigue, and irritability.

It is not possible to say exactly how large a supplement is required to cause an overdose. One person might develop toxic symptoms from the same dose that another can tolerate.

Nonetheless, I have combed through scientific reports trying to get an idea of the level needed to cause side effects. Among adults, it seems that the lowest amount linked to overdoses is about 300 IU per pound of body weight.

In other words, an adult weighing 100 pounds might overdose after taking a supplement of 30,000 IU on a regular basis. A 150-pound adult might have a toxic reaction to a dose of 45,000 IU. Symptoms usually do not develop for months or years.

Reports of toxic effects usually involve higher doses. But to be cautious, several scientific committees have warned against adult doses higher than 25,000 IU per day, except when severe deficiency of vitamin A exists. Children and infants, of course, cannot tolerate nearly as much as adults.

When overdosages do occur, the symptoms usually subside shortly after the offending pills are stopped.

I did learn of one case, though, where a young boy required a year to recover fully.

Of course, if your doctor has prescribed vitamin A supplements for you, that is another story. High doses of vitamin A supplements have been used to treat some skin disorders, such as psoriasis—that's how we learned of the side effects. By all means, follow your doctor's advice if these supplements are prescribed.

Can You Eat Too Much Vitamin A?

The vitamin A in animal foods can cause over-dosages, too. But about the only way to get an overdose from food is to eat lots of liver. There are stories of vitamin A overdosages in arctic explorers who ate polar bear liver. It has more vitamin A than most of us eat in a week.

Of course, supermarkets don't sell polar bear liver. Of the commonly available forms, beef liver is highest in vitamin A. In fact, it has about five times the vitamin A of chicken liver and four times that of pork liver. The U.S. Department of Agriculture (USDA) has found, however, that the vitamin A content of all liver varies widely within each class.

To give you an idea of how much liver would be expected to cause an overdose, I've calculated how much of each type would provide 50,000 IU of vitamin A. If consumed daily, or almost daily, such a level might pose a risk to the average adult. Few people, however, eat liver on such a frequent basis.

Nonetheless, here are the amounts of liver that supply about 50,000 IU of vitamin A:

- 1 slice of beef liver (6½ by 2½ inches)
- 16 chicken livers (2 by 2 inches)

- 3 cups chicken liver, chopped
- 1¾ slices pork liver (6½ by 2½ inches per slice)

The Real Problem with Animal Sources

Aside from liver, overdosing on other animal foods that have vitamin A is difficult—if not impossible. But there are other reasons not to depend on animal foods for most of your vitamin A. First, it is not clear whether this kind of vitamin A has any value in preventing cancer.

As mentioned earlier, some studies link only the carotene form of vitamin A to protection from cancer. But in the case of stomach cancer, there are studies linking milk consumption with reduced chances of getting the disease. Because milk contains vitamin A, this suggests a possible role for animal vitamin A in cancer prevention.

But many animal foods with vitamin A have serious drawbacks. Let's take a look at them:

- Butter contains vitamin A but also high levels of saturated fat and calories. Use it in small amounts, or substitute margarine. Margarine has the same calorie and fat count, but the fat is mostly unsaturated.
- Whole milk and whole milk cheeses are good sources of vitamin A but also have a high fat and calorie count. Use part-skim cheeses when you can, and eat cheeses in small amounts. Drink skim or low-fat milk; both have as much vitamin A as whole milk but less fat and calories.
- Egg yolk provides vitamin A but is also high in cholesterol. Try to eat only three per week.
- Liver is rich in vitamin A but, like egg yolk, is

high in cholesterol. Eat it infrequently or in small amounts.

Beef, lamb, and pork have modest amounts of vitamin A, but some cuts are high in fat and calories. Choose the leanest cuts, and trim away as much fat as possible.

Some fish are also modest sources of vitamin A. Herring, salmon, and sardines fall into this category. These fish also contain higher levels of fat than most fish, though the fat is unsaturated. Always drain and rinse them well if packed in oil. Chub and pink salmon have less fat (and less vitamin A) than the red variety.

A Change in Measurement of Vitamin A

One final note about vitamin A. Nutritionists are changing to a new methods of measuring this nutrient.

Until recently, vitamin A was measured in IU. Food manufacturers who give nutrition information for their products still express vitamin A content in this way.

In the future, however, you probably will see vitamin A listed in a different way. The new measurement is called retinol equivalents, and it is often abbreviated as RE.

For most of us, this change means getting used to small numbers. One retinol equivalent is the same as 3.33 IU vitamin A from the animal form (retinol). For carotene, one retinol equivalent is the same as 10 IU. A food that has 1000 IU of carotene has only 100 RE.

The RDA for vitamin A is 5000 IU for men. In retinol equivalents, the RDA is a smaller number: 1000 RE.

Most food tables have not been updated yet; they still list vitamin A in IU. For this reason, I have had to use IU when describing the vitamin A content of foods.

Actually, there is little reason for you to be converting IU of vitamin A into RE. It doesn't matter if you think of vitamin A in foods as IU, RE, or simply as low, medium, and high—as long as you make sure to get your fair share.

4

Vitamin C

Focus on this chapter if you smoke cigarettes *and* drink alcohol, work with hazardous chemicals, or eat large amounts of cured or pickled foods. If your doctor has told you that you have a premalignant condition of the esophagus, ask for personalized dietary advice on a regular basis.

It is time to rewrite our nutrition textbooks.

The textbooks of yesterday tell us that vitamin C prevents scurvy. They talk of the vitamin's role in healing wounds. They explain that vitamin C aids in the formation of collagen, which holds cells together.

But an update is in order.

It's not that vitamin C does not do these things. Rather, it does more—much more.

It may very well help to prevent cancer, says the Committee on Diet, Nutrition, and Cancer.

The panel members were impressed enough with studies of vitamin C and cancer to advise us to eat foods rich in vitamin C every day.

At the federal government's National Cancer Institute, the view is no different. In 1977, the institute advised the public to eat "ample amounts of fruits and vegetables." Fruits and vegetables, of course, provide most of our vitamin C.

Scientists have found that cancers of the stomach and esophagus are less common among people who eat diets rich in vitamin C. In fact, year-round access to foods rich in vitamin C may be one explanation for the dramatic fall in stomach cancer rates in the United States.

Stomach cancer was common in the United States at the turn of the century, when some fruits and vegetables were available only seasonally. We now have year-round access to these fruits and vegetables, and many are rich in vitamin C. And stomach cancer is no longer common here. It does remain a major health problem in some parts of the world.

A few studies also tie vitamin C to lower risk of bladder and colon cancer. But there is not enough research yet to make a firm judgment about vitamin C's ability to protect against these two forms of cancer.

How Vitamin C Protects Us

We have a pretty good idea of how vitamin C works to prevent cancer. As you probably have read, substances in food called nitrites can turn into cancer-causing nitrosamines during cooking or digestion. Bacon, of course, has a particularly bad record; nitrosamines have often been found in it after cooking.

Laboratory scientists know that nitrosamines can be created by letting certain chemicals come in contact with each other. Yet when vitamin C is added to the chemical mixture that normally results in nitrosamines, fewer of them form. In some cases, vitamin C has completely blocked the formation of nitrosamines.

Can the same thing happen in our bodies? Studies around the globe suggest that the answer is yes.

Here in the United States, a team of researchers found that the chances of developing cancer of the esophagus went down as the amount of fruits and vegetables in the diet went up. Researchers also know that Americans and Western Europeans have fairly low rates of stomach cancer. These countries enjoy access to a variety of fruits and vegetables.

On the other hand, fruit and vegetable intake is low in some of the regions where stomach and esophageal cancer are rampant. Iranians living along the coast of the Caspian Sea, for instance, have alarming rates of esophageal cancer. Researchers sent to find out why noted that fruits and vegetables were almost absent from the diets of these people.

Another Role for Vitamin C

Scientists have known for decades that vitamin C can block the chemical reaction called oxidation. Oxidation is the process that causes food to become rancid. Substances that prevent oxidation are called antioxidants.

Until recently, no one realized that antioxidants might help protect against cancer. But they very well may. Scientists now believe that some chemicals cause cancer only if oxidized. By preventing oxidation, vitamin C may cut down on our exposure to cancer-causing chemicals.

The Recommendation
and How to Meet It

"Eat fruits, vegetables...daily, especially those high in vitamin C," advises the Committee on Diet, Nutrition, and Cancer. This is going to be a popular recommendation. Almost everyone—from babies to adults—likes foods rich in vitamin C.

To follow the committee's advice, take a look at the following chart. It rates foods as low, medium, or high in this vitamin. Animal foods are not listed because they supply less than 10 percent of the vitamin C in the American diet. Fruits and vegetables are the foods to depend on for this nutrient.

Vitamin C in Fruits and Vegetables

Low*	Medium**	High***
Apples	Apricots	Asparagus
Celery	Bananas	Broccoli
Cucumber	Beets	Brussels sprouts
Grapes	Blackberries	Cabbage
Pears	Carrots	Cantaloupe
Plums	Cherries	Cauliflower
Pumpkins	Corn	Grapefruit
	Dark green leafy	Green pepper
	vegetables	Kohlrabi
	Kale	Lemons
	Mangoes	Limes
	Peaches	Oranges
	Potatoes (white)	Peas
	Spinach	Pineapple
	Summer squash	Raspberries
	Watermelon	Strawberries
	Winter squash	Sweet potatoes
		Tangerines
		Tomatoes

  * Low: Less than 5 milligrams (mg) per average serving.
  ** Medium: 5 to 20 mg per average serving.
*** High: More than 20 mg per average serving.
Adapted from the work of Committee on Diet, Nutrition, and Cancer, National Academy of Sciences, 1982.

How Much Is Enough?

Again, the Committee on Diet, Nutrition, and Cancer did not tell us how much vitamin C to take in every day. The RDA for vitamin C is 60 mg a day for adults. By the way, 60 mg of pure vitamin C crystals would measure only a fraction of a teaspoon.

The scientists who set the RDA, however, did not take the evidence on vitamin C and cancer into account.

Here is some more specific advice. Nutritionists have always recommended four or more servings a day of fruits and vegetables. I think at least two, and preferably three, should be foods supplying moderate to high amounts of vitamin C. I try to eat a food rich in vitamin C at every meal.

It is not hard. I can hardly start the day without my orange juice. So this is my first suggestion. Grapefruit juice is also a fine choice.

Here are some other tips that work for me:

- Top cereal with sliced peaches, bananas, or other foods that are good sources of vitamin C.
- Eat salads often, using deep green lettuce, green pepper, and tomato as ingredients.
- Add sliced peaches to chicken salad.
- Serve luncheon salads inside of fresh green peppers.
- Serve fruit for dessert. If the family objects, make sweets that include fruit. It is simple enough to top cakes or ice milk with sliced bananas, berries, peaches, or other fruit.

If you are wondering what qualifies as a serving, here are some guidelines. For juices, three-fourths to one cup is one serving. "Juice" glasses usually hold three-fourths of a cup (6 ounces). Full-size glasses usually hold a full cup (8 ounces).

Nutritionists generally consider three-fourths of a cup of a vegetable as one serving. If that doesn't mean much to you, take a look at half cup and quarter cup measures to get an idea of what three-fourths of a cup looks like.

For most fruits, such as oranges, bananas, or apples, one whole fruit is one serving. For large fruits such as grapefruit, half of one fruit is one serving. In the case of very large fruits, such as melons, you can consider one cup of the fruit, diced, as one serving.

Vitamins A and C Often Go Hand in Hand

If it seems that eating to prevent cancer is getting complicated, rest assured that it does not have to be.

When it comes to eating more of the fruits and vegetables rich in vitamins A and C, you can often get both nutrients from the same foods. There are quite a few foods that are good sources of both of these important nutrients.

You might call them the fruit and vegetable all-stars. Here is the lineup:

- Asparagus, broccoli, cantaloupe, sweet potatoes, and tomatoes are high in both vitamins A and C.
- Brussels sprouts, green pepper, and peas are rich in vitamin C and also contain moderate amounts of vitamin A.
- Apricots, mangoes, mixed vegetables, peaches, romaine lettuce, spinach, and winter squash have medium amounts of vitamin C and high levels of vitamin A.

- Dark green leafy vegetables, such as kale, collards, and turnip and mustard greens are also rich in vitamin A, with moderate amounts of vitamin C.
- Corn, green beans, and watermelon have moderate amounts of both vitamins A and C.

One nice aspect of vitamins and cancer is that many of these foods complement each other in cooking. Sometimes I mix apricot nectar with orange juice to give a not-too-sweet breakfast beverage. That way I start my day right, with both vitamins A and C.

As you read through the recipe section, you will find many tasty ways to combine these foods, making it easy to meet the recommendations for both vitamins A and C.

By the way, I cannot resist pointing out that most of these foods rich in vitamins A and C are pleasantly low in calories, too.

Handle with Care

Vitamin C is very sensitive. Heat, light, and oxygen can do it in. In fact, some loss of the vitamin C in food just cannot be prevented.

With a little effort, though, losses of the vitamin can be kept to a minimum.

Here are the rules:

- The sooner fresh foods can be used, the better. Vitamin C breaks down during storage.
- Try not to chop these foods finely all the time. The fewer pieces a food is cut into, the lower its exposure to oxygen, which destroys vitamin C.
- The vitamin C in cabbage, cantaloupe, squashes, and strawberries is especially unstable. The sooner they are eaten after cutting, the better.

- When using water to cook foods rich in vitamin C, boil the water first. Then add the food and cover the pot tightly. This cuts down on the oxygen coming in contact with the food.
- Cook vitamin C–containing foods in as little water as possible. The vitamin can leach into the cooking water. Steaming in a basket or pressure-cooking is better, because less liquid will come into contact with the food.
- If you do cook these foods in water, use the cooking water to make a sauce or save it for stock. This way, you won't pour vitamin C down the drain.
- Keep cooking time to a minimum. The longer the food is cooked, the more vitamin C it will lose.

It is not always possible, of course, to follow these rules, but when it is, do so. The vitamin will also hold up better if not heavily exposed to light.

About Frozen Foods

All of this talk about losing vitamin C must make you wonder if any of it is left in processed foods. The answer is: it depends.

In some cases, the ability of the food industry to preserve the vitamin C in food is no less than amazing. In other instances, though, it seems that processors are not trying hard enough.

My favorite example is frozen orange juice concentrate. It contains hardly a milligram less vitamin C than the oranges that it hails from. The juice processors have perfected their trade so well that it is almost an art.

Many other frozen foods do lose some vitamin C

during the trip from field to supermarket. But their fresh counterparts are likely to do so, too, during storage and cooking. So, though fresh, raw vegetables usually have the most vitamin C, once cooked, their C content may be on a par with that of frozen foods.

If you observe the rules on preserving the vitamin C in foods, your fresh, cooked vegetables may retain more vitamin C than frozen ones.

Is There Vitamin C in That Can?

For canned fruits and vegetables, the story is not so good. Canned foods often have less vitamin C than frozen or fresh foods. The vitamin C leaches into the water used in packing.

So even though a canned food might have a lower cost per pound than the fresh or frozen version of the same item, it is not necessarily the best buy. If the canned version has only half as much vitamin C as the frozen, for instance, it actually can cost more to get 20 milligrams of vitamin C from it.

I do not want to imply that canned foods have no nutritional value. Nor do I mean to say that canned foods should never be used. But nutritionally, frozen foods are often a better buy. When in season, fresh foods are often a better buy, too. And fresh or frozen foods usually have less salt—a big plus.

You almost always can depend on fresh, uncooked foods for vitamin C (provided that the food is a source of the vitamin). When you eat fresh, raw foods, you don't have to give a thought to losses that occur during cooking.

To give you an idea of how cooking affects vitamin C, I've put together the following chart.

The Vanishing Vitamin
Vitamin C Lost during Cooking and Storage

Green Beans		Peas	
1 cup, raw	21 mg	1 cup, raw	39 mg
1 cup, fresh, cooked*	13–15 mg	1 cup, fresh, cooked*	32 mg
1 cup, frozen, cooked*	7 mg	1 cup, frozen, cooked*	21 mg
1 cup, canned	5 mg	1 cup, canned	14 mg

*Boiled just until tender, in a small to moderate amount of water.

Remember: the vitamin C that remains in frozen or fresh foods can be destroyed by too much exposure to heat, light, and large amounts of cooking liquid. But a little effort can go a long way toward preventing unnecessary losses of this important vitamin.

Best Buys for Vitamin C

As I said earlier, I am one of the original bargain-hunters. But I have high standards for my bargains. Quality counts just as much as the price tag.

I have taken a close look at fruits and vegetables to figure out how to get the most vitamin C for my money.

I did the same thing for foods high in vitamin C that I did for those that provide vitamin A. I picked a fixed amount of vitamin C, amounting to ⅓ of the RDA. I then calculated the cost of getting this amount of vitamin C (20 mg) from an array of fruits and vegetables. I examined fresh, frozen, and canned.

Here is what I have learned:

• Grapefruit juice, orange juice, raw broccoli, and raw green peppers are best buys. They provide 20 mg of vitamin C for four cents or less.

- Other popular foods that are also a great buy are tomato juice, oranges, frozen broccoli, and fresh cabbage.
- Strawberries and cantaloupe can be good buys for vitamin C—when they are in season.
- Brussels sprouts, cauliflower, and dark green leafy vegetables also rate high when cost per 20 mg of vitamin C is calculated.

For those who want the whole story, the following chart tells it. Note that the amount of food needed to provide 20 mg of vitamin C is also listed.

Getting Your Money's Worth
Cost of 20 mg Vitamin C from Fruits and Vegetables

2¢: Grapefruit juice, frozen concentrate, ¼ cup, prepared
4¢: Orange juice, any form, ¼ cup
    Broccoli, fresh, ⅛ cup
    Green pepper, raw, 2 tablespoons, chopped; ¼ medium pepper
    Grapefruit juice, canned, ¼ cup
6¢: Broccoli, frozen, ¼ cup
    Brussels sprouts, frozen; ¼ cup
    Collards, frozen, ⅓ cup
8–10¢: Oranges, fresh, ⅓ fruit
    Cabbage, fresh, ½ cup
    Strawberries, fresh, ¼ cup
    Tomato juice, canned, ½ cup
    Cauliflower, frozen, ¼ cup
12–14¢: Grapefruit, fresh, ¼ fruit
    Lemon, fresh, ½ medium
    Cantaloupe, fresh, ⅓ cup, diced
    Limes, fresh, 1 medium
    Turnip greens, canned, ½ cup
    Strawberries, frozen, ⅛ cup
    Spinach, frozen, ½ cup
    French fries, frozen, 16 medium strips

Getting Your Money's Worth (continued)
Cost of 20 mg Vitamin C from Fruits and Vegetables

16–19¢: Papaya, fresh, ⅛ fruit
         Spinach, fresh, ⅔ cup, raw
         Yellow summer squash, fresh, 1 cup, sliced or
            diced
         White potatoes, fresh, 1 medium round
         Spinach, canned, ⅔ cup
         Tomatoes, canned, ½ cup
         Peas, frozen, 1 cup
20–29¢: Tomato, fresh, 1 medium
         Watermelon, fresh, 2 cups, diced
         Mango, fresh, ⅓ cup, diced
         Sweet potatoes, canned, ⅔ cup, pieces
         Peas, canned, 1½ cups
         Zucchini, fresh, 1¼ cups, sliced, cooked
         Sweet potatoes, fresh, 1 medium
30–40¢: Banana, fresh, 1½ large or 2 small
         Nectarine, fresh, 1
         Carrots, fresh, 3 7-inch
         Romaine lettuce, fresh, 2 cups, raw
         Pineapple, canned, 1 cup
         Corn, canned, 2 cups

Calculations are based on July 1982 prices in a Washington, D.C., supermarket. Vegetables are assumed to be cooked unless otherwise noted. A 30 percent loss of vitamin C has been deducted for fresh, cooked vegetables because of losses likely to occur during cooking.

A Word to Smokers

Smokers—take notice of three important facts:

• Smokers have less vitamin C in their blood than nonsmokers.

- Smoking combined with drinking raises the risk of mouth and esophageal cancers.
- Vitamin C is linked to reduced chances of getting these cancers.

I cannot tell you why, but repeated studies have shown that smokers have anywhere from 30 to 50 percent less vitamin C in their blood than nonsmokers. And it is not because smokers take in less vitamin C. They get as much of the vitamin as nonsmokers.

For years we have known that the amount of vitamin C in the blood decreases with age. But a recent study found that smokers aged twenty to thirty-nine had less vitamin C in their blood than nonsmokers aged forty to sixty-four.

When I read about these findings I thought that the smokers might be excreting more vitamin C, rather than putting it in their blood. But this doesn't seem likely. Scientists trying to figure out what's happening have found that the smokers do not excrete more vitamin C than nonsmokers. On the contrary—they excrete less.

Apparently, smokers are using up more of the vitamin C they take in. The smoker's body may be using extra vitamin C in an effort to counteract the harmful substances in tobacco smoke.

Whatever the reason, it makes good sense for smokers to ensure a good intake of vitamin C.

If you have more than two or three drinks a day and smoke as well, you should pay even closer attention to your vitamin C intake. Those who smoke *and* drink heavily have a much higher risk of mouth and esophageal cancer. Since vitamin C is linked to lower rates of these two cancers, this is another reason for those who smoke and drink to include more vitamin C in their diets.

The Controversy
over Vitamin C Supplements

The Committee on Diet, Nutrition, and Cancer took a stand against the use of vitamin C supplements to meet its recommendations.

I think that scientists who take this position have one of two reasons. One is a very good one. But the other, in my opinion, is not so good.

The studies that tie vitamin C to cancer prevention usually link *foods containing vitamin C* rather than the vitamin itself to reduced risk of cancer. There is always the possibility that it is something else in these foods, rather than the vitamin C, that is protecting our health. If this is the case, people who take a vitamin C pill rather than eat vitamin C–containing foods will miss that unknown protective substance. Personally, I think that it is probably the vitamin C itself that is protective, though I also believe that other substances in these same foods have anti-cancer ability.

Of course, ideally we should get our vitamin C from foods. But some people just don't care for vegetables, which supply almost 40 percent of the vitamin C in the American diet. And some parents have tried, but failed, to convince their children to eat more fresh fruits and vegetables.

I simply cannot see withholding a moderate vitamin C supplement when this is the case. I think it is unscientific to advocate a diet that contains 200 mg of vitamin C a day, yet oppose a supplement of this amount for those people who do not eat foods rich in vitamin C.

In my field there is a long history of opposition to vitamin supplements. Unfortunately, it has become an automatic response among some nutritionists. I cannot go along with it though, because sometimes it doesn't make sense.

Can It Hurt?

For all the noise that has been made about vitamin C supplements, you would think there were dead bodies lined up next to bottles of vitamin C.

When I was a graduate student, I decided that I did not want to swallow the anti-vitamin dogma without taking a close look at the research myself. Fortunately for me, my university granted me credit for an independent study project on this subject. I spent an entire semester researching the benefits and hazards of high doses of certain nutrients. It was an education in itself.

I went to the finest medical library in the country, the National Library of Medicine, and used its computer to search out every reported case of adverse reactions to four vitamins. I learned that in high doses some nutrients can cause more side effects than some drugs. At high doses, a vitamin such as nicotinic acid (a version of the vitamin known as niacin) really is a drug. But when it came to vitamin C, the research led me in a different direction. Try as I might, I could only conclude that vitamin C was one of the least toxic substances in the pharmacy.

First, I would like to tell you that, in general, the amount of vitamin C that has been reported to cause problems in some people is far beyond the level you would get by eating a diet rich in fruits and vegetables. But even at high doses, toxic effects appear to be the exception rather than the rule.

But I would like to mention four problems that have been linked to very high doses of vitamin C:

- kidney stones and aggravation of gout
- destruction of vitamin B-12
- complications from lack of the enzyme G6PD
- interactions with prescription drugs

The Kidney Connection

It is true that high doses of vitamin C may speed formation of kidney stones. This side effect may occur mostly among people who are especially prone to kidney stones. Remember, though, that not everyone who tends to develop kidney stones knows it.

How much vitamin C did it take to bring on kidney stones or the early signs of stones? According to a commentary published in the *New England Journal of Medicine,* this problem has been seen in people taking four or more grams of vitamin C every day.

The same process that makes kidney stones more likely to form may also worsen gout. People who are susceptible to gout should also take note of these findings.

About Destruction of Vitamin B-12

It is also possible, but probably not likely, that vitamin C may destroy some of the vitamin B-12 in food.

A few years ago, two scientists put together some laboratory equipment to mimic digestion. They reported that under these "test-tube" conditions, a 500 mg supplement of vitamin C destroyed a high percentage of the vitamin B-12 in food.

When another scientist directly studied this issue in human subjects, the results were different. This researcher examined vitamin B-12 levels in the blood of people who had been taking at least 500 mg of vitamin C daily. He found that only three of the ninety people tested had low levels of vitamin B-12. These three, all fifty to sixty years of age, had been taking a minimum of 1000 mg of vitamin C with each meal for more than three years.

There is one more fact to note regarding the effect of vitamin C on vitamin B-12. Scientists believe that less B-12 will be destroyed if the vitamin C is taken two or more hours after eating.

If You Have G6PD Deficiency

I found one death linked to high doses of vitamin C. "High dose" is actually an understatement. This case involved a man who had been given 80 grams of vitamin C for two days as a treatment for burns. He died a few weeks later.

It turned out that this patient had a deficiency of the enzyme G6PD. The abbreviation G6PD stands for glucose-6-phosphate dehydrogenase. As its name implies, this enzyme is used in metabolism of glucose, a type of sugar.

Although this man had been given an enormous amount of vitamin C, scientists are concerned that others with G6PD deficiency may be sensitive to smaller amounts. If you have this condition, you should be aware of this concern.

About 10 percent of black American males have mild G6PD deficiency. A smaller percentage of black females are affected, as are a few Caucasians. Screening tests for this condition are readily available.

Mixing Vitamin C
with Prescription Drugs

If you take any of the following prescription drugs, consult your physician before taking a vitamin C supplement.

- warfarin sodium
- dicumarol
- tricyclic antidepressants
- amphetamines

Pharmacologists have expressed concern that vitamin C may occasionally interfere with the action of these drugs. Pregnant women, also, should take only as much vitamin C as prescribed by their physicians.

Beyond the Cancer Question

I would drink my orange juice and eat my green peppers even if it weren't for research linking vitamin C to prevention of cancer.

Some of my reasons are the same ones that bolster the advice to eat more fruits and vegetables that supply carotene. Like these plant foods rich in vitamin A, foods rich in vitamin C are also low in saturated fat and sodium.

What's more, fruits and vegetables that contain vitamin C are cholesterol-free. And they provide small to moderate amounts of dietary fiber. Eaten in large amounts, the fiber in these fruits and vegetables helps to lower blood cholesterol levels.

There is more. Vitamin C is rarely recognized for its role in iron absorption. Yet we have known for many years that vitamin C helps the body to absorb iron.

The extent of iron deficiency in the United States has been greatly exaggerated, I believe, but there are probably more Americans taking in too little iron than is the case for other nutrients.

Because the body absorbs only about 10 percent of the iron taken in, factors that increase iron absorption are just as important as iron-rich foods. In fact, some scientists believe that increasing absorption of iron, rather than boosting iron intake, is the key to improving iron nutrition. They may be right on target.

At moderate levels—such as 50 to 100 mg—vitamin C has been found to improve iron absorption by as much as 50 percent. Higher doses may result in even higher absorption. But very few of us truly need such an assist.

Vitamin C helps the body absorb iron in foods that are eaten *at the same meal.* The vitamin C in breakfast foods, for example, has little or no effect on the iron in foods eaten at lunch or dinner.

For some people, however, this is not good news. A small number of people have a condition that causes them to retain too much iron, which accumulates in various organs, causing health problems. People who have this condition should consult their physicians for advice about diet.

I would love to tell you that vitamin C will also help protect you from heart disease. But I cannot, because I am not at all convinced by these claims.

I have looked carefully at evidence that vitamin C lowers blood cholesterol levels. But I found other studies in which vitamin C supplements appeared to have raised the cholesterol level. Some studies show no difference. I really do not hold out much hope for an effect here.

But what more can you want from vitamin C? It

does not have to play a role in prevention of every disease in order to be taken seriously.

In my opinion, vitamin C is as important today as it was two centuries ago, when the mysterious disease called scurvy threatened the lives of sailors who spent months without fresh fruits and vegetables. It is hard to disagree with the advice to make more room for this familiar vitamin in our diets.

5

Dietary Fiber

Focus on this chapter if you eat large amounts of meat or high-fat foods. If your doctor has told you that you have ulcerative colitis or intestinal polyps, you are at higher risk of developing colon cancer. Ask for personalized dietary advice on a regular basis.

In the history of nutrition, there never has been a story quite like that of dietary fiber.

For decades, nutritionists viewed fiber as all but worthless. It did not even qualify as a nutrient, because its absence didn't cause the deficiency diseases that result when diets are inadequate in protein, vitamins, or minerals.

As far as nutritionists could see, fiber served no useful purpose other than to prevent constipation.

But during the past decade, fiber has come into its own. It is now the focus of intense research. It is now known that fiber plays a role in regulation of blood cholesterol and blood sugar. Fiber may even help with weight control.

And, yes, it is likely that fiber can help to prevent cancer. The Committee on Diet, Nutrition, and Cancer has advised us to eat whole grain foods *every day*. These foods are usually a good source of fiber.

61

Grains that have been refined—such as white flour—contain less fiber.

The Fiber Fan Club

The Committee on Diet, Nutrition, and Cancer was not the first to recommend more fiber-containing foods. In 1980, the USDA issued new dietary guidelines. USDA now recommends eating "foods with adequate starch and fiber."

This was quite a change for the USDA. For twenty-five years, its food guides made no distinction between refined grains and whole grains; both were considered about equal in nutritional value.

And back in 1977, when the National Cancer Institute issued its advice to the public, it, too, advocated eating more fiber.

The average American eats about 20 grams of fiber per day. Several scientists have recommended increasing fiber intake to a level of 30 to 40 grams a day. You will find several charts in this chapter that will enable you to determine how your fiber intake compares to the recommended level.

Fiber: What It Is

Fiber is a general term. It refers to an assortment of substances in food that are not digested in the small intestine. With one exception, all forms of fiber are carbohydrates. They are a type of carbohydrate that humans cannot digest.

All of the following are classified as dietary fiber:

• cellulose, which is abundant in wheat bran
• hemicelluloses, another form found in whole grain foods

- lignin, found in grains, fruits, and vegetables
- pectins, which are common in fruits and vegetables
- gums and mucilages, often found in beans, oats, fruits, and vegetables.

The Two Basic Types of Fiber

Actually, you don't have to know each form of fiber and where it occurs. For the most part, it is only necessary to think of two kinds of fiber: soluble and insoluble.

As their label implies, the soluble fibers are those that dissolve in water. Pectins, gums, and mucilages fall into the soluble category.

Insoluble fibers are those that do not dissolve in water. Cellulose, hemicelluloses, and lignin are insoluble fibers.

Both soluble and insoluble forms of fiber play important roles in preventive medicine. *Current research suggests, however, that only the insoluble fibers help to prevent cancer.*

The insoluble fibers create bulk in the digestive tract. The more bulk there is, the less room for harmful chemicals that might cause cancer. The soluble fibers do not give bulk, but they do have other virtues. We'll talk about them later in this chapter.

The best source of the bulk-producing insoluble fibers is whole grain foods—especially bran.

Studies worldwide link whole grain foods to lower risk of colon cancer. Studies on animals back up these results. In animals, wheat bran has more often than not shown an ability to help protect against colon cancer.

A few studies with humans have also tied vegetables to low rates of colon cancer. The fiber in vegetables has rarely been tested in animals, however, so it is hard to pass judgment on foods other than whole grains.

It is no surprise, then, that the Committee on Diet, Nutrition, and Cancer limited its advice on fiber to whole grain foods.

The Recommendation and How to Meet It

None of the recommendations from the Committee on Diet, Nutrition, and Cancer are as simple as the one for fiber. "Eat...whole grain foods daily," advises the panel.

In providing fiber, no whole grain food comes close to wheat bran. Half a cup of 100 percent whole bran cereal has about three times as much fiber as a slice of whole wheat bread.

You don't have to eat bran directly to add it to your diet, though starting the day with a bran cereal is not a bad idea. You can replace a small amount of flour used in baking with bran. Because bran is so rich in fiber, even a small amount counts. As a general rule, try replacing about one-third of the flour in a recipe with an equal amount of bran.

When baking with bran cereal, it is best to let the cereal soften in liquid before baking. Try to combine the cereal with a liquid ingredient in the recipe.

Be Creative with Cereals

Shredded wheat is another excellent source of wheat fiber. Many people find the "spoon-size" shredded wheat more pleasing than the large biscuits.

There are dozens of ways to enjoy shredded wheat:

- Use the spoon-size biscuits with dips.
- Crush the biscuits with a rolling pin and substitute for some of the flour used in baking.
- Use spoon-size biscuits with soups and salads instead of croutons. You may want to sauté them first in a small amount of margarine or butter for about five minutes.
- Substitute spoon-size shredded wheat for rice when serving a meat or vegetable sauce that is normally served over rice. The liquid in the sauce will soften the cereal, as is the case for the High-Fiber Chow Mein in the recipe section.

Some of the "chex" cereals are also a good source of fiber. Bran Chex has the most fiber of the group. Wheat Chex also provides some fiber; it is made with the whole grain. The corn and rice varieties are made from refined grains. Their fiber content is negligible.

The chex cereals make a good breakfast cereal for those who like crunchy cereal. Shredded wheat tends to soften quickly when milk is added.

Another delicious use for the chex cereals is in party mixes. Mixed with chopped dried fruit and popcorn, this is my choice for a great snack. See My Favorite Munch in the recipe section.

Oats are still another versatile whole grain food. Instant oats, quick oats, and old-fashioned oats are all whole grain foods. The difference lies in the way the oats are cut. The instant oats are steamed at the factory. Unlike quick or old-fashioned oats, instant oats contain added sodium.

Hot cereal is the most obvious use for oats, but there are many other ways to enjoy them.

- Favor recipes calling for oats in baked goods such as cookies.

- Use oats instead of white bread in meat loaf and other recipes where bread serves as a meat extender.
- Use an oat crust instead of cracker crust in baking pies. See the recipe section for directions.

Choosing Your Morning Menu

Probably the simplest way to add whole grain fiber to your diet is to choose a whole grain cereal for breakfast. The chart that follows classifies common breakfast cereals based on their content of whole grains. Because the sugar content of cereals is important to many people, it, too, is rated.

Two stars in the "Whole Grain" column signals a product made exclusively with whole grains or bran. One star indicates that the cereal is partially whole grain. Cereals made only with refined grains have no stars. The far right column shows the sugar content. Cereals that contain very little or no sugar (less than 2 grams per serving) have been awarded two stars. Those with a moderate sugar content (3 to 9 grams per serving) earn one star. High-sugar cereals have no stars in this column.

Rating the Cereals

Cereal name	Whole grain	Sugar
All-Bran (Kellogg)	**	*
Bran Buds (Kellogg)	**	*
Bran Chex (Ralston)	*	*
Corn Flakes (Kellogg)		**
Cracklin' Bran (Kellogg)	**	*
Cream of Wheat, plain (Nabisco)	**	**
C. W. Post Granola (Post)	**	*
Frosted Flakes (Kellogg)		

continued on page 67

Rating the Cereals (continued)

Cereal name	Whole grain	Sugar
Fruit 'n Fibre (Post)	*	*
Grapenuts (Post)	**	**
Heartland (Pet)	**	*
Life (Quaker)	*	*
Nature Valley Granola (General Mills)	**	*
—Nutri-grain (Kellogg)	**	**
Oats: Quick or Old-Fashioned or plain Instant (Quaker)	**	**
100% Bran (Nabisco)	**	*
100% Natural (Quaker)	**	*
Product 19 (Kellogg)	*	**
Puffed Wheat or Rice (Quaker)		**
Ralston (Ralston)	**	**
—Shredded Wheat (Nabisco, Quaker)	**	**
Special K (Kellogg)	*	**
Total (General Mills)	**	**
Wheaties (General Mills)	**	**

More Whole Grain Ideas

Of course, there are whole grain foods other than those that we think of as cereals.

Here are some ideas for whole grain foods that go well with lunch and dinner or make good snacks:

- for lunch: whole wheat or rye bread
- for dinner: brown rice, millet, bulghur wheat (as in tabouli)
- for snacks: graham crackers, rye wafers, or whole wheat crackers

All of these foods are moderate sources of insoluble fiber.

A Matter of Milling

You may be surprised to see brown rice and whole wheat bread described as only moderate sources of fiber. These foods contain less fiber than is commonly believed.

Brown rice, for example, has only a moderately higher fiber content than white rice. The difference amounts to about 1½ grams per half cup of cooked rice.

Whole wheat bread has more fiber than brown rice, yet less than many people assume. It is a moderate source of fiber, but not one of the highest. In general, coarse wheat products have more fiber than breads.

There is another reason why coarse forms of wheat, such as bran and shredded wheat, are better sources of fiber than foods such as whole wheat bread. The beneficial effects of these fiber-containing foods is partly due to the bulk they create in the digestive system.

Grinding wheat into flour reduces its ability to create bulk in the digestive tract. A finely ground source of fiber—such as whole wheat bread—does not give as much bulk as bran.

Because of this, foods made from whole grain flour do not have as much laxative power as bran and other coarse forms of wheat. It is possible that foods made from finely ground whole grains also have less value in preventing cancer.

Baking with Fiber

Baking with whole wheat flour instead of white is another way to boost your fiber intake. In yeast breads, making this substitution poses no problem.

But baking cakes and cookies with whole wheat flour increases the amount of fat needed for good texture. Cakes and cookies made with whole wheat flour require about one and one-half to twice as much fat as those made with white flour. And some people find their heavy texture unappealing.

One way to solve this problem is to use half white flour, and half whole wheat flour when baking. This should hold down the amount of fat needed.

If you are interested in the extra minerals in whole grain flour, rather than its small amount of fiber, there is another option. Use a quarter of a cup of wheat germ and three-quarters of a cup of white flour for each cup of flour in a recipe. You'll get roughly the same nutrients as in whole wheat flour, with the exception of its fiber.

The Penny-Pincher's Guide

One thing is for sure: following the recommendation to eat whole grains is not going to break your budget. Many whole grain foods are reasonably priced.

I have computed the cost of getting a gram of fiber from an assortment of common foods. Here is what I learned:

- Unprocessed bran is the cheapest source of fiber. Each gram costs less than a penny.
- The bran-only cereals such as All-Bran and 100%

Bran also provide a gram of fiber for only a penny.

- Store-brand whole wheat and rye bread give a gram of fiber for just over a penny.

If you like unprocessed bran, it may actually be a better buy at a health food store, where it is sometimes sold in bulk rather than in fancy packages. My own taste buds prefer bran muffins baked with the bran-only cereals. But I have included some recipes using the unprocessed bran because it is a little less expensive.

Individually packed instant oats and a few cereals are expensive ways to get whole grain nutrition. But most of the cereals are reasonably priced, and boxed oats are a good value.

Here is the price tally for whole grains:

Fiber for Pennies
Cost of a Gram of Fiber from Foods

1¢: Unprocessed bran, 1 teaspoon
All-Bran cereal (K), 2 teaspoons
100% Bran cereal (N), 1 tablespoon
Whole wheat bread (S), ½ slice
Rye bread (S), ½ slice

2¢: Bran Chex cereal (R), 2 tablespoons
Corn Bran cereal (Q), 2 tablespoons
Spoon-size Shredded Wheat, 3 tablespoons
40% Bran cereal (K,P), 3 tablespoons
Old-Fashioned Oats (Q), 2 tablespoons, uncooked
Quick Oats (Q,S), 2 tablespoons, uncooked
Whole wheat bread (S), ½ slice

3¢: Most cereal (K), 2 tablespoons
Raisin Bran cereal (K,S), 3 tablespoons

4¢: Wheat Chex cereal (R), ⅓ cup
Rye wafers, 1⅓ triple cracker

continued on page 71

Fiber for Pennies (continued)
Cost of a Gram of Fiber from Foods

5¢ or more: Instant oats (Q), ⅓ packet Wheaties or Total cereal (G), ½ cup

Letters in parentheses stand for manufacturer: Kellogg (K), Ralston (R), General Mills (G), Quaker (Q), Post (P), store brand (S).

More Foods with Fiber

Fiber comes in other foods, too. As I said earlier, the Committee on Diet, Nutrition, and Cancer made recommendations only for whole grains. But I would like to mention some other sources of fiber that have the bulk-producing ability of the whole grains.

Among beans, fruits, and vegetables, the best sources of insoluble fiber are:

- kidney beans and white beans
- peas
- blackberries
- parsnips

I have learned to use peas in both hot and cold recipes; I add them to meat dishes and stews as well as to salads. I have also found that for a change of pace, beans make a nice salad. The Bean and Artichoke Salad in the recipe section is one of my favorites.

The following foods have less insoluble fiber than the above foods. But they still have respectable amounts:

- apples, pears, plums, and strawberries
- lima, pinto, or green beans
- broccoli and brussels sprouts
- potatoes (white)
- summer squash, tomatoes, and zucchini

Animal foods, fats, and oils contain no fiber. Only plant foods have it.

How Much Is Enough?

It makes good sense to eat more whole grain foods and more fiber. As mentioned earlier, a fiber intake of 30 to 40 grams has been proposed by several experts.

This does not mean that all the grains in your diet must be whole grains, or that every fruit and vegetable you choose must rate high for fiber.

My advice is to make about half the grains in your diet whole grains. I am not with those who despise any grain food made from refined grains.

True, refined grain foods contain less of certain minerals than whole grain foods. And they have less fiber, though in some cases (such as brown versus white rice or whole wheat pasta versus white pasta), the differences are small.

But this is not to say that foods made with white flour are worthless. They provide respectable levels of protein, iron, and certain vitamins. And they are low in fat and cholesterol and often low in sodium.

In short, there is something good to be said for both whole grain and refined grain foods. A reasonable balance between the two is a moderate, sensible approach.

If you want to estimate your fiber intake, consult the charts that follow. The first gives the total fiber content of foods. The remaining two divide fiber into the two basic types: insoluble and soluble.

Total Fiber Content of Foods
(Soluble and Insoluble)

1 gram

Almonds, 10
Apricots, 2 medium
Asparagus, ½ cup
Banana, 1 small
Bean sprouts, ½ cup
Bread, white, 1 slice
Bread, french, 1 slice
Cauliflower, ½ cup
Cherries, 10
Cucumber, raw, ½ cup
Egg noodles, cooked, ½ cup
Eggplant, ½ cup
Graham crackers, 2
Grapefruit, ½
Kale, ½ cup
Lettuce, raw, ½ cup
Peach, 1 medium
Peanuts, 10
Pecans, 2
Pineapple, ½ cup
Rice, brown, ½ cup
Roll, dinner, 1
Spaghetti, ½ cup
Turnips, ½ cup

2 grams

Brussels sprouts, ½ cup
Carrots, ½ cup
Corn grits, cooked, ½ cup
Oats, cooked, ½ cup
Onions, ½ cup
Rutabagas, ½ cup
Strawberries, ½ cup
Green beans, ½ cup

continued on page 74

Total Fiber Content of Foods (continued)
(Soluble and Insoluble)

2 grams

Summer squash, ½ cup
Tomatoes, ½ cup

3 grams

Bread, rye, 1 slice
Bread, whole wheat, 1 slice
Broccoli, ½ cup
Pear, 1 small
Popcorn, popped, 3 cups
Zucchini, ½ cup

4 grams

Apple, 1 small
Beans, kidney, ½ cup
Beans, white, ½ cup
Blackberries, ½ cup
Parsnips, ½ cup
Potato, 1 small

5 grams or more

All-Bran cereal, ½ cup
Bran Buds cereal, ½ cup
100% Bran cereal, ½ cup
Grapenuts cereal, ½ cup
Peas, ½ cup
Rolled oats, dry, ½ cup
Shredded wheat cereal, 2 large biscuits

Unless otherwise indicated, all values for vegetables reflect fiber content of the cooked product. Analyses of fiber content by James W. Anderson, High Carbohydrate and Fiber Research Foundation, Lexington, Kentucky.

Insoluble Fiber Content of Foods

Low*	Medium**	High***
Apricots, 2 medium	Apple, 1 small	Beans, kidney, ½ cup
Asparagus, ½ cup	Beans, lima ½ cup	Beans, white, ½ cup
Banana, 1 small	Beans, pinto, ½ cup	Blackberries, ½ cup
Bean sprouts, ½ cup	Beans, green, ½ cup	100% Bran cereal, ½ cup
Bread, French, 1 slice	Bread, rye, 1 slice	Parsnips, ½ cup
Bread, white, 1 slice	Bread, whole grain, 1 slice	Peas, ½ cup
Beets, ½ cup	Broccoli, ½ cup	Shredded Wheat, 2 large biscuits
Carrots, ½ cup	Brussels sprouts, ½ cup	
Cauliflower, ½ cup	Corn grits, ½ cup	
Cherries, 10	Graham crackers, 2	
Cucumber, ½ cup, raw	Oats, whole, ½ cup	
Egg noodles, ½ cup	Pear, 1 small	
Eggplant, ½ cup	Plums, 2 small	
Grapefruit, ½	Popcorn, popped, 3 cups	
Grapes, 10	Potato, 1 small	
Kale, ½ cup	Rice, brown, ½ cup	
Lettuce, raw, ½ cup	Rye wafers, 3	
Onions, ½ cup	Strawberries, ¾ cup	
Peach, 1 small	Tomatoes, ½ cup	
Pineapple, ½ cup	Whole wheat cereal flakes, ¾ cup	
Radishes, raw, ½ cup	Zucchini, ½ cup	
Rice, white, ½ cup		
Roll, dinner, 1		
Rutabagas, ½ cup		
Spaghetti, ½ cup		
Tangerine, 1 medium		
Turnip, 1 medium		

  * Low: less than 1 gram
 ** Medium: 1 to 2.9 grams
*** High: 3 grams or more

Unless otherwise indicated, all values for vegetables and pasta reflect fiber content of the cooked product. Values determined by James W. Anderson, High Carbohydrate and Fiber Research Foundation, Lexington, Kentucky.

Soluble Fiber Content of Foods

Low*	Medium**	High***
Asparagus, ½ cup	Apricots, 2 medium	Apple, 1 small
Beans: kidney, lima, white, ½ cup	Banana, 1 small	Broccoli, ½ cup
	Beans, green, ½ cup	Carrots ½ cup
Bean sprouts, raw, ½ cup	Beets, ½ cup	Peas, ½ cup
	Blackberries, ½ cup	Plums, 2 small
Bread, French, 1 slice	Brussels sprouts, ½ cup	Potato, 1 small
#Bran, ½ cup	Corn grits, ½ cup	Summer squash, ½ cup
Cauliflower, ½ cup	Eggplant, ½ cup	Tangerine, 1 medium
Cherries, 10	Grapefruit, ½	Zucchini, ½ cup
Cucumber, raw, ½ cup	Kale, ½ cup	
Grapes, 10	Onions, ½ cup	
Lettuce, raw, ½ cup	Pear, 1 small	
Oats, whole, ½ cup	Popcorn, popped, 3 cups	
Parsnips, ½ cup	Rutabagas, ½ cup	
Peach, 1 medium	Strawberries, ¾ cup	
Pineapple, ½ cup	Tomatoes, ½ cup	
Radishes, raw, ½ cup	Turnips, ½ cup	

* Low: 0.5 gram or less
** Medium: 0.6 to 1.0 gram
*** High: 1.1 grams or more
#Other wheat products such as whole wheat or white bread, pasta, and graham crackers are insignificant sources of soluble fiber. Brown and white rice also contain very little soluble fiber.

Unless otherwise indicated, classification of vegetables is based on values for the cooked products. Analyses of fiber content done by James W. Anderson, High Carbohydrate and Fiber Research Foundation, Lexington, Kentucky.

Can Fiber Cause Trouble?

There is one reason not to go all out when it comes to fiber. Though it has its good points, fiber has not been given a clean bill of health just yet.

Nutritionists have known for decades that fiber

can bind to minerals in food, preventing the body from absorbing them. All forms of fiber have this ability.

Scientists believe that we may be able to adapt to high-fiber diets. But this is not known for sure. It is speculation based on a handful of studies.

The effect of fiber on minerals varies among the different types. Here is what scientists think based on current knowledge:

- Iron nutrition probably won't be affected by eating more fiber.
- Fiber probably will decrease absorption of zinc and copper.
- If zinc and copper intake is good, the decrease in absorption probably will not create any problems.

Whole grains contain more zinc and copper than refined grains, so this may offset any loss of these minerals resulting from the fiber. But until we know this for a fact, I feel it's best to take a moderate rather than extreme approach to the fiber content of your diet.

Another Mineral-Robber

Fiber is not the only substance in whole grain foods that can bind to minerals. Whole grains also contain phytic acid, which can also tie up minerals. Nutritionists also refer to phytic acid as phytate.

Fortunately, we now know that yeast can destroy phytate. This means that it should not be a problem in whole grain breads made with yeast.

Nutritionists believe that phytate is rarely a problem, except among people eating enormous amounts of unleavened bread. Few, if any, Americans eat such a diet.

Fighting Fat with Fiber

If you're a weight watcher, you probably remember the "starch blockers" that came out in 1982. The too-good-to-be-true claims were just that. The pills landed more than two dozen people in the hospital. The Food and Drug Administration had its hands full getting the stuff off the market.

Well, fiber may be the only starch blocker that doesn't make us sick.

Nutritionists have long known that fiber blocks the absorption of some of the calories in food. It not only blocks the calories from carbohydrates; it takes on protein, fat, and carbohydrate pretty much equally. Studies show that people absorb 1 to 3 percent fewer calories when eating a high-fiber diet.

Sound like a fantasy? It is not. Most of us gain weight slowly, at the rate of an extra pound or two per year. For a woman needing 1800 calories a day, a 1 percent fall in calories absorbed would mean a loss of two pounds per year. A 3 percent reduction in calories absorbed translates into six fewer pounds per year.

There's only one catch. These findings come from short-term studies. No one knows whether the body will adapt to a high-fiber diet so that eventually just as many calories are absorbed.

Fiber researchers have reported getting complaints from their subjects about the "large" quantity of food they were asked to eat. Little did the subjects realize that the high-fiber diets contained no more calories than the low-fiber diet.

This is a clue that fiber creates a feeling of fullness. Nutritionists have long suspected that it does. In the stomach, fiber swells with water. This may help curb hunger.

Some scientists also believe that high-fiber foods help with weight control because they take longer to chew.

One thing is for sure: a high-fiber diet based on whole grains, fruits, and vegetables is likely to be nutritionally sound. That is more than can be said for so many of the "miracle" weight-loss diets that come along every year.

More Benefits of Fiber

Fiber is now known to benefit the following conditions:

- diverticulosis and diverticulitis
- high blood cholesterol
- diabetes

It may also help prevent tooth decay!

Let's take a closer look at these findings.

Diverticulosis is a common condition among older Americans. It refers to outpouchings of the intestines. Food can get caught in these pockets. Often the result is inflammation and pain.

Doctors used to treat this problem with a low-fiber diet. But much to their surprise, they have learned that a high-fiber diet usually gives much better results. In general, patients are asked to add wheat bran to their diets.

Dental researchers believe that whole grain foods may play a role in preventing tooth decay. Studies show that something in whole grains may protect the teeth from decay-producing acids in the mouth. The bacteria in the mouth produce these acids.

Two More Feathers in Fiber's Cap

The soluble forms of fiber have value in control of blood cholesterol and blood sugar. Fruits, vegetables, beans, and oat bran are good sources of these forms of fiber.

The soluble fibers don't lower blood cholesterol nearly as much as saturated fats and cholesterol raise it. But a diet rich in fruits and vegetables has a mild cholesterol-lowering effect, thanks to the fiber. Lower blood cholesterol, of course, means lower rates of heart disease.

These soluble forms of fiber have also revolutionized the treatment of diabetes. New research has shown that a high-fiber diet helps diabetics control their blood sugar better than the diets used in the past. Their insulin requirements often drop on a high-fiber diet. *Changes in insulin doses should be made only on a doctor's instructions.*

Fiber's ability to keep the blood sugar under control may very well help people who do not have diabetes. A low-fiber meal can cause the blood sugar level to rise quickly, then drop abruptly. Headaches, hunger, and irritability can set in as a result.

But fiber can guard against these symptoms by preventing sharp swings in the blood sugar level.

If you would like detailed information on the soluble fiber content of foods, see the chart that appeared earlier in this chapter. For more information about fiber, see the Further Readings section.

6
Cancer Inhibitors in Food

Focus on this chapter if you often eat foods that are pickled, cured, or high in fat. If your doctor has told you that you have ulcerative colitis or intestinal polyps, you are at higher risk of developing colon cancer. Ask for personalized dietary advice on a regular basis.

Do you think of cancer as a mighty sword that can reach down and hurt any and all of us? At any time?

If you do, then you should think again. Exciting new research shows that nature gives us weapons that can fight back. And these weapons are not in exotic places. They are in common foods.

I am not talking now about the nutrients you have read about in earlier chapters. The substances I'm talking about are not considered nutrients, because their absence does not cause a deficiency disease. These substances are little-known food elements. Only a handful of research scientists are familiar with them.

Scientists call them inhibitors. In laboratory animals, these substances show an impressive ability to inhibit the cancer process.

How Cancer Inhibitors Work

A cancer agent, such as one found in cigarette smoke, might cause cancer in half of the animals that are exposed to it. But when an inhibitor is given along with the cancer-causing chemical, fewer animals will develop cancer. The inhibitor prevents the cancer-causing chemical from doing its damage.

Exactly how inhibitors work is not known. But the best theory right now has to do with an enzyme system in the body's cells. It is called the mixed function oxidase system. Scientists believe that this enzyme system may actually have the power to strip dangerous chemicals of their harmful effects.

Cancer scientists have been curious about inhibitors for a very good reason. *Human studies do support the notion that certain foods help to block the cancer process.* Several studies have found that people who often eat foods thought to contain inhibitors have less chance of getting cancer.

The Organs That Benefit

For the most part, inhibitors are linked to protection against cancer of the digestive organs. Research ties these inhibitors most strongly to reduced rates of stomach and colon cancer.

Cancer inhibitors may help to explain why many people who are exposed to cancer agents never develop cancer. Think about it. Everyone has been exposed to cancer agents. They are in the air. Or in the water we drink. Or in the workplace. And sometimes in our food.

Why, then, does cancer strike one in four—not four in four?

A good intake of cancer inhibitors may be part of the answer.

The Recommendation and How to Meet It

The Committee on Diet, Nutrition, and Cancer took a close look at research on cancer inhibitors. The committee made one recommendation after looking at these important findings.

The recommendation advises us to emphasize foods belonging to the cabbage family of vegetables. There is good evidence that these foods contain cancer inhibitors other than vitamins A and C.

The most common foods of the cabbage family are broccoli, cauliflower, brussels sprouts, and, of course, cabbage. Research has linked these four vegetables to reduced risk of both stomach and colon cancer. A few studies also link these foods to lower risk of rectal cancer.

There are other foods in this family of vegetables. But it is not possible to say whether these other foods are also linked to lower risk of these cancers. It is reasonable to believe that these other foods are more likely than not to contain the same cancer-blocking substances. But only further research will give a firm answer.

The following chart lists all the foods belonging to this family.

The Whole Cabbage Family

Broccoli	Collards	Mustard
Brussels sprouts	Horseradish	Radish
Cabbage	Kale	Rutabaga
Cauliflower	Kohlrabi	Turnip
Chinese cabbage	Kraut	Watercress

A Family of Many Names

Scientists have some strange jargon for the foods of the cabbage family. The most technical name for this group of foods is the *Brassica* family. If you hear this term, just think cabbage family. Scientists also refer to these foods as "cruciferous" vegetables.

The inhibitors found in broccoli, brussels sprouts, cauliflower, and cabbage have been named indoles.

Research on indoles is so recent that tables listing the indole content of foods are nowhere to be found. So it is not possible to rank foods by their indole level. Also it is not known whether cooking and storage influences the indoles in these foods.

The best advice is to select the foods of this family that you like best and eat them often—perhaps once or twice a week. Remember that many of these foods offer other bonuses: vitamins A or C, a low fat and sodium count, and a modest amount of dietary fiber.

Putting Cabbage on the Menu

This is quite a family of foods. Some of these foods are as versatile as a vegetable can be. They can start out in soup or salad. They can take the form of a side dish. Or they can star in the main course.

Other family members, though, are suitable only for a specific dish. And some are only condiments.

The stand-out family member is broccoli. It's awarded "favorite vegetable" status by many people.

If you like raw broccoli, you can use it with dips and on salads. You can add it to soups—leave it in pieces or purée it. Try adding curry powder to the soup.

In the recipe section, you can find some broccoli side dishes, as well as main dishes using this vegetable.

Cauliflower can be used in all of these ways, too. And broccoli and cauliflower go well together in both side dishes and main courses.

Cabbage, of course, can be used in salad or soup. The recipe section gives recipes for cole slaw and spicy cabbage soup. Cabbage can be added to main dishes such as chili or stir-fried with apples and onions for a great side dish. The recipe section gives samples for these uses, too.

Brussels sprouts are not quite as versatile—or as popular. This vegetable is best suited as a side dish, though I have seen it stuffed with cheese as an appetizer.

Two members of the cabbage family—radish and watercress—are used mostly as salad ingredients. But I have encountered both in soups, too. Another family member—the turnip—can replace potatoes in many recipes. The greens in this family—collards, kale, and mustard greens—work best as a vegetable side dish.

Cabbage Cookery

If you are not familiar with some of these vegetables, you may be interested in the following guidelines for preparing them:

- Do not remove the outer leaves of broccoli, cabbage, cauliflower, and brussels sprouts until you are ready to cook them.
- Thick stems of broccoli can be cut in half, lengthwise, for cooking.
- Cauliflower can be cooked whole or cut into flowerets.

- Cut a head of cabbage into quarters for cooking—unless shredding it for a salad or recipe. When using a food processor, shred cabbage with the *slicing* blade. The shredding blade will chop it too fine.
- Remove base of raw brussels sprouts before cooking.
- To retain vitamin C, steam these vegetables or prepare in a pressure cooker. Use of a microwave oven also helps retain nutrients.

Cooking Times for the Cabbage Family

Cooking times for these vegetables depends on several factors, such as their size and age. Here are some rough estimates for boiling or steaming these vegetables when raw.

- broccoli: 20-25 minutes
- cauliflower, cut into flowerets: 10-15 minutes
- mustard or collard greens: 5-15 minutes
- brussels sprouts: 10-20 minutes
- cabbage (cut into fourths), turnips, kale, or whole cauliflower: 20-30 minutes
- kohlrabi: 20-40 minutes
- cabbage, shredded: 8-12 minutes

Remember: the sooner these vegetables are prepared after purchase, the more nutritious they will be.

Other Foods That May Help

The cabbage family is not the only group of foods that has shown potential to block the cancer process.

Other foods may also have this ability—and some may be even more potent than foods of the cabbage family.

But the evidence for these other foods is not as strong. Some foods have inhibited cancer in studies on animals, but studies with humans have yet to be done. Other foods have been studied in only one or two experiments—too few for judgment.

This is why the Committee on Diet, Nutrition, and Cancer limited its recommendations to the cabbage family.

Of the other foods that might also contain inhibitors, the evidence is best for citrus fruits. The beneficial effect of these foods has ranged from weak to potent in studies with animals.

As for other foods, the evidence is just beginning to come in. But for your information, I would like you to know some of the possibilities now under further study:

- Celery and spinach have shown slight but significant inhibiting ability.
- Soybeans and lima beans have also shown some potential.
- Grains and vegetable oils may contain a substance with moderate inhibiting power.
- Green coffee beans have shown a powerful inhibiting effect in early studies. But roasted and instant coffee have shown only a weak effect.

Remember: for some of these foods only one or two studies have been done. This is far too little work to justify changing your diet.

Some Unanswered Questions

Scientists are still a little cautious about the cancer inhibitors in food. They aren't 100 percent convinced that these substances are only beneficial.

The Committee on Diet, Nutrition, and Cancer tells us that it's a matter of weighing the pluses and minuses. On the balance, the panel scientists agreed that the good points of the cabbage family vegetables outweigh the bad points.

What are the bad points? Mostly, they fall under the label of "uncertain effects."

As noted earlier, inhibitors seem to activate an enzyme system that is thought to detoxify harmful chemicals. There is some concern that this very same enzyme system may also enhance the power of some chemicals. In other words, the enzyme system may have both good and bad effects.

"Information on this subject is incomplete," says the Committee on Diet, Nutrition, and Cancer. Still, the scientists recommend that we eat citrus fruits, whole grains, and cabbage family vegetables. Obviously, the scientists think that the pluses here outweigh the minuses.

But until this question is settled, it is best not to go all out with cabbage family vegetables. Eating them often—but not exclusively—is probably the best course of action. Including them in your diet once or twice a week is a cautious, moderate approach.

Putting It All Together

Up to this point, you have read a great deal about fruits, vegetables, and grains. But this chapter is the last one that involves these foods directly.

It is fitting, I think, to take a broad look at these foods to see how they score when all protective factors are taken into account.

There are four factors to consider: vitamin A, vitamin C, insoluble fiber, and inhibitors. To take a simple approach to these four factors, I have devised a rating system.

I gave a food one point if it contains a moderate amount of vitamin A and two points for a high level. I used the same system for vitamin C and for insoluble fiber.

I then awarded two points to the four members of the cabbage family that appear to contain a cancer inhibitor other than vitamins A and C or fiber. I gave one point to the other foods that might have a cancer inhibitor.

The Top-Scoring Foods

When all the points were tallied, broccoli and brussels sprouts topped the list.

They were followed by some vegetables that many people eat little of: collards, kale, kohlrabi, mustard greens, and rutabagas.

But in third place were some familiar faces: oranges, grapefruit, cabbage, cauliflower, lima beans, and spinach. Watercress also rated with this group.

Chances are that you like some of these foods. Pick the ones you like best, and continue to enjoy them.

7

Minerals

Wouldn't it be great to have a "quick fix" for every disease—a pill that would prevent or cure all health problems? No one would have to give a thought to diet, exercise, or other health habits.

It is an alluring idea. Some have even proposed that the quick fix already does exist—in the form of a mineral called selenium.

But the wishful thinking is a little premature. There is some evidence that the minerals in our food play a role in preventing cancer. More research is needed, though, before we can draw any conclusions.

The Minerals in Food

Food contains a wide range of minerals. We need some of them in large amounts. Other minerals are required in very small amounts.

Nutritionists refer to the minerals needed in large amounts as major minerals. Those that we need in small amounts are known as trace minerals or trace elements.

The most important major minerals are

- calcium
- magnesium

- sodium
- chloride
- phosphorous
- potassium

There are many trace minerals. Scientists know a great deal about some of them, and very little about others. Some of the trace minerals include

- copper
- chromium
- fluorine
- iodine
- iron
- manganese
- molybdenum
- selenium
- zinc

When it comes to minerals and cancer, research has focused only on trace minerals. None of the major minerals have been the focus of cancer research.

Too Soon to Tell

The Committee on Diet, Nutrition, and Cancer made no recommendations about minerals. In general, the scientists found too little evidence for making judgment.

The panel members cited selenium and iron as the best-studied minerals. But though they found evidence that selenium may protect both humans and animals against some forms of cancer, the evidence was ruled preliminary.

Similarly, the committee members found evidence that an adequate iron intake protects both humans and animals against cancer in the upper part of the digestive tract. But these findings, too, were considered inconclusive.

The committee said that no conclusions could be drawn at all about the role of the following minerals in cancer prevention:

- copper
- zinc
- molybdenum
- iodine
- arsenic
- cadmium
- lead

It may surprise you to read the committee's conclusions about these last three minerals—arsenic, cadmium, and lead. You may be aware that these minerals have long been linked to excessive cancer rates among workers who are heavily exposed to them. But occupational exposure to these minerals is many times higher than the levels that occur in food. For this reason, too, the committee declined to make any judgments.

The Selenium Story

Chances are that you have heard reports about the ability of selenium to prevent cancer. A few enthused promoters have inspired some people to take selenium supplements as a preventive measure.

The evidence that selenium helps to prevent cancer is promising but far from final. Research has shown, for instance, that

- Areas of the world where selenium intake is high have lower cancer rates than countries where the diet is low in selenium.
- Blood selenium levels are higher in healthy people than in cancer victims.
- Selenium added to the diet or drinking water of laboratory animals helps to protect against cancer-causing chemicals.

One problem with these findings is clear. Scientists can rarely know whether a cancer patient always had a low blood level of selenium. It is possible that the disease, once developed, caused a normal selenium level to drop suddenly.

Some research has yielded opposite results, showing no relationship between the selenium in the blood and the risk of cancer. But on the whole, the research on this mineral must be considered promising.

Oddly enough, there were once concerns that selenium might promote cancer. These fears have not been supported by the most recent research.

But research has shown that selenium can be toxic in other ways. Scientists hardly want to advocate a measure that will help prevent one disease but cause others instead.

Be Careful with Supplements

Encouraged by reports linking the mineral to cancer protection, people are buying—and taking—selenium supplements. But a few words of caution are in order.

At high doses, selenium can cause health problems. Fatigue and irritability, as well as brittleness or loss of hair, have been seen in patients suffering from toxic amounts of selenium. A research scientist exposed to too much selenium developed bronchitis and skin problems.

How Much Is Too Much?

According to the Food and Nutrition Board of the National Research Council, a long-term intake of 2400 to 3000 micrograms of selenium per day would be expected to cause a toxic reaction.

It is very unlikely that the diet could provide such a high level of selenium. In fact, there is only one recorded instance of selenium toxicity caused by food. It dates back about fifty years and occurred among people living in an area of the country where the soil was unusually rich in this mineral.

To overdose on selenium, you would probably have to work with it or take supplements. In 1977, the Food and Nutrition Board advised:

There is no justification at this time for the use of selenium supplements by the general population. Should selenium supplements eventually be considered desirable for those persons living in low-selenium areas, or for those consuming vegetarian diets, *a daily supplement of 50 to 100 micrograms could probably be taken safely.* (Emphasis added.)

Five years later, in 1982, the Committee on Diet, Nutrition, and Cancer seemed to agree with the Food and Nutrition Board's opinion. "Increasing the selenium intake to more than 200 micrograms a day . . . by the use of supplements has not been shown to confer health benefits exceeding those derived from consumption of a balanced diet," said the panel.

Selenium in Our Diet

It is not easy to list the selenium content of common foods. The amount of selenium in meat, for instance, can vary. It depends partly on the amount of the mineral in the animals' diets.

The selenium content of the soil also varies throughout the regions of the United States. The soil content, in turn, greatly affects the amount of selenium in grains. But most Americans now eat foods grown from many parts of the country; no longer do we eat only foods grown nearby.

As a result, nutritionists rarely see signs of selenium deficiency among Americans. The average selenium intake in the United States is 150 micrograms per day, which is considered more than enough for most people.

Good sources of selenium are

- meat and seafood
- grains, unless grown in soil low in selenium
- asparagus and mushrooms
- garlic

Meats and seafood are the richest source of this mineral.

Fruits and most vegetables contain little selenium. The selenium content of dairy products and eggs varies.

Can Iron Help, Too?

Adequate iron in the diet prevents a condition called Plummer-Vinson syndrome. This condition has been linked to increased risk of developing stomach cancer and cancer of the esophagus.

Probing these findings, scientists have found that iron deficiency allows bacteria to grow in the stomach. It is possible that these bacteria turn nitrites into the cancer-causing substances called nitrosamines.

But, as is the case with selenium, there is still not much evidence to go on. It certainly makes sense, though, to eat iron-rich foods (unless your doctor has advised against it. Some people, though not many, have a disorder that causes them to retain too much iron).

Iron deficiency is not truly widespread in the United States. But many Americans don't get the RDA for iron. This hardly means that all of these people have iron deficiency. The RDA is set higher than about 96 percent of us need. It is not a requirement, but rather a "better-safe-than-sorry" approach.

The Best Sources of Iron

If you are concerned about your iron intake, consider some of these sources:

- lean meats and shellfish
- whole grain or enriched cereals
- dried apricots, prunes, or raisins
- nuts and wheat germ
- dried beans and peas
- leafy green vegetables

Liver, especially pork liver, contains large amounts of iron. But it is also rich in cholesterol. Too many of us eat too much of cholesterol-containing foods. Egg yolk has a moderate iron content; it, too, is high in cholesterol.

The iron in flesh foods, called heme iron, is best absorbed by the body. Yet studies have found no more iron-deficiency anemia among vegetarians than among meat-eaters.

One possible explanation is vitamin C. It enhances absorption of the iron in foods. Vegetarians often consume more vitamin C than meat-eaters. The vitamin C may compensate for the absence of meat in their diets.

A Look at Lead

Lead has long been in the headlines. Lead poisoning has occurred too frequently among children—often from eating chips of old paint that contained lead.

Whether lead also plays any role in the cancer process is an open question. Only a few studies have been done—mostly in animals. These studies suggest that large amounts of lead might increase the risk of kidney cancer. But this form of cancer is not very common.

The Committee on Diet, Nutrition, and Cancer declined to make any recommendations regarding lead.

Some Advice Nonetheless

Lead remains a concern to health experts for other reasons. The chances of getting lead poisoning are not great, but the problem has yet to be eliminated in this country. Infants, children, and pregnant women are at greater risk.

Scientists estimate that food accounts for 55-85 percent of our exposure to lead. The lead in canned foods can seep into the food itself. Public pressure and encouragement from the Food and Drug Administration have led canners to reduce the lead content of food by almost 40 percent during the last four years.

Acidic foods packed in cans made with lead are the most likely to absorb this mineral. Fruits and fruit juices, including tomato products, fall into this category. If these foods are stored in the can after opening, the lead content can increase fivefold in less than a week.

Lead experts urge us not to store acidic foods in cans after opening. Transfer the food to a glass or plastic container. This precaution will go a long way to preventing unnecessary lead in the diet. Foods taste better, too, when this advice is followed.

Unfortunately, there is no easy way to tell whether a can has been soldered with lead. Evaporated milk is usually packed in lead-soldered cans. Infant formulas are not. Processed meats are also usually packed in nonleaded cans.

There's Much More to the Story

Though research has yet to find that lead or other minerals play a major role in cancer prevention, the story of nutrition and cancer is not yet over. We have looked at vitamins, minerals, fiber, and cancer inhibitors. But there's more to come.

The next chapter tells about the dietary change that may offer the biggest dividends of all.

8

Dietary Fat

Focus on this chapter if you eat few foods rich in fiber or few foods of the cabbage family. If there is a history of breast, ovary, or prostate cancer in your family, or if you were or will be thirty-five or older at first pregnancy, you should also read this chapter carefully.

It is a shame that so many people believe that eating less fat means eating less flavor. First, in the opinion of this nutritionist, this isn't necessarily so. And second, there is probably no dietary change that will do more for your health.

You probably know that eating less fat is the most important step in reducing your calorie intake. No doubt you also know that eating less saturated fat is the key to preventing heart disease through diet.

These two facts alone are reason enough for eating less fat. But there is more.

According to the Committee on Diet, Nutrition, and Cancer, eating less fat is the best thing you can do to beat the odds of developing cancer.

"Among the dietary factors we examined, a linkage between total fat consumption and colon, breast, and prostate cancer stands out most prominently," explains Dr. Clifford Grobstein, chairman of the committee.

99

A Clear Case for Cutting Down

Grobstein and his fellow committee members did not have to search high and low for evidence linking low-fat diets to low risk of getting these forms of cancer. There is plenty of it—and it comes from all corners of the globe.

What makes the case for eating less fat so convincing?

First, the simple fact that many nations have very low rates of breast, colon, and prostate cancer is pretty good evidence that these cancers don't have to happen. If the people of some nations can grow old with little chance of getting these cancers, it is obvious that *they can be prevented*.

Research spanning forty countries makes clear that these three forms of cancer are rare where diets are low in fat. So are cancers of the ovary and uterus. Scientists have also found that as people give up low-fat diets, they increase their risk of these forms of cancer. Migrants from Japan, for instance, who traditionally ate diets very low in fat, began to lose their low risk of these diseases after living in the United States. Today, Japanese-Americans born in the United States have the same high risk of breast cancer as the general population.

Research on animals confirms that diets lower in fat do help to prevent cancer. In fact, this finding is not new. As long ago as 1930, scientists found that low-fat diets helped prevent breast cancer in animals. Intense research during the past ten years shows that low-fat diets also help prevent colon cancer in laboratory animals.

How Low Fat Diets Protect Us

Scientists have a good hunch about how fat affects our risk of developing breast cancer. Apparently, fat in the diet can affect a woman's hormone levels. These hormone levels, in turn, seem to influence the development of breast cancer. *Current theory holds that when little fat is eaten, the hormone pattern is affected in a way that gives breast cancer much less chance of growing.*

Similarly, fat in the diet probably affects men's hormone levels. *Again, when the diet is low in fat, the hormone pattern is unfavorable to the growth of prostate cancer.*

And when we watch our fat intake, conditions in the digestive tract discourage the growth of colon cancer. The reason? To digest fat, the body produces substances called bile acids. The less fat you eat, the fewer bile acids you have.

Scientists think that the bile acids—or at least some of them—encourage the growth of colon cancer.

I agree with those who say that you have nothing to lose by eating less fat—except pounds. Now let's talk about how to do it.

How Fat Is Measured

Before looking at the recommendation on fat, it is important to know how fat intake is measured.

There are several ways to measure the fat in your diet. Nutritionists feel that the most meaningful is the *percent of calories* method.

Fat is one of the few substances in food that provides calories. Aside from fat, the only other food elements that give calories are:

- protein
- carbohydrate
- alcohol

The percent of calories from fat simply tells us the proportion of the day's calories that fat is providing. If fat provides 20 percent of the calories in your diet, the remaining 80 percent is coming from protein and carbohydrates and, possibly, from alcohol.

In the average American diet, fat provides a whopping 40 percent of calories. Needless to say, that is too much.

The Recommendation and How to Meet It.

Though the average fat intake in the United States is too high, few health professionals advocate going to the opposite extreme. *The recommendation is to lower fat intake to provide no more than 30 percent of the day's calories.* This level has been endorsed by the Committee on Diet, Nutrition, and Cancer and the Senate Select Committee on Nutrition and Human Needs.

There are dozens of ways to make this recommendation. What's more, scientists have tested the practical side of this advice. They have shown that a diet containing 30 percent of calories from fat does taste good enough to eat!

Only Four Basic Guidelines

You can meet the 30 percent fat guideline by following only a few ground rules (we will look at them in greater detail in the rest of this chapter):

- Low-fat milk products are emphasized.

- Only lean meats, poultry, and fish are used.
- Cooking and table fats (butter, oil, and margarine) are used in moderation—about one pat (roughly one teaspoon) of margarine per slice of bread or serving of vegetables.
- Bread, pasta, cereal, fruits, and vegetables are emphasized.

An Alternative: The Gram-Counting Method

If you have long been a calorie-counter, you may prefer a different approach to watching your fat intake. This method involves counting the grams of fat in your food. I don't mean counting every gram of fat every day. Rather, I suggest doing it for a week or two to get an idea of the foods that will help you cut your fat intake.

To use the gram-counting method of watching your fat intake, you need a rough idea of your ideal calorie intake. Once you know that, you can easily figure out how many grams of fat to allow yourself each day.

To save you the arithmetic, I have made the calculations myself. If, for instance, you need only 1000 calories per day, eating 33 grams of fat per day will keep your fat intake at the recommended level of 30 percent of calories.

Here is the maximum recommended fat intake for other common calorie levels:

- 1200 calories: 40 grams of fat
- 1500 calories: 50 grams of fat
- 1800 calories: 60 grams of fat
- 2000 calories: 67 grams of fat
- 2400 calories: 80 grams of fat
- 3000 calories: 100 grams of fat

Books listing the grams of fat in common and brand name foods can be found in bookstores. See the Appendix for information on obtaining one of these books.

The Best of the Dairy Case

No doubt about it, there are some terrific dairy foods. They not only provide reasonable levels of fat and calories but also calcium, protein, and certain B-vitamins.

The top-ranking dairy foods include

- skim or low-fat milk
- low-fat yogurt
- low-fat cottage cheese, although regular cottage cheese (4 percent fat) is not bad

In addition, some brands of ice milk contain little fat. These brands, along with some other frozen dairy foods, offer a low-fat alternative to ice cream. Buttermilk contains a fair amount of salt but is usually made with low-fat milk. It, too, is welcome on a low-fat diet.

Using Dairy Beverages

As is the case for all dietary changes, the switch from high-fat to low-fat dairy products should be made gradually. Overnight changes are not likely to become lifetime habits.

There are obvious and not-so-obvious ways to use low-fat dairy beverages in your diet. Here are some suggestions:

- Use skim or low-fat milk in cooking as well as at the table.
- Use buttermilk instead of whole milk in baked goods and pancakes.
- To thicken skim milk used in cooking, add a little nonfat milk powder.
- Use evaporated skim milk in baked goods calling for evaporated milk.

You can save money by making your own "evaporated skim milk." Start with nonfat dry milk and add only half as much water as needed to make skim milk.

Cottage Cheese and Yogurt Ideas

I will be the first to admit that I don't like cottage cheese—as is. But I use at least a pound a week. Here is why:

- A cup of cottage cheese, two tablespoons of skim milk, and a tablespoon of lemon juice whipped in a blender provides a tasty, low-fat alternative to sour cream.
- Some of my favorite pancake recipes call for cottage cheese—see the recipe section for details.
- Cottage cheese can often replace about half of the high-fat hard cheese in casseroles.

I also don't care for plain yogurt—but my grocery bills show that I use plenty of it. I use only yogurt labeled *low-fat*. Several brands contain whole milk—and almost twice as much fat as the low-fat varieties. Here is where all the yogurt goes in my household:

- into the blender, accompanied by fruit, to make terrific "shakes" (see recipe section)

- into a paper coffee filter, which I leave in the plastic dripping cone over a mug in the refrigerator; in a half day or so I have a tasty "yogurt cheese" as good as high-fat cream cheese
- into a dipping bowl, mixed with garlic, onion, and other spices to make a light and low-fat dip
- into salads where I once used high-fat, high-calorie mayonnaise
- into salad dressings, particularly those seasoned with dill or traditionally made with mayonnaise

Yogurt, by the way, substitutes well for buttermilk in baked goods.

Low-Fat Dairy Treats

I rarely eat ice cream. I don't miss it because the grocery store is filled with tasty low-fat alternatives.

The fat content of ice milk varies because states impose their own rules for the fat content. Some brands of ice milk have very little fat, while others have almost as much as ice cream. From the standpoint of taste, many leave much to be desired.

Surveys rating ice milk have found, however, that one brand—Kraft's Light 'n Lively—is excellent in taste. It also has the lowest fat content permitted by federal law: only one-third as much fat as in most brands of ice cream.

Other frozen low-fat desserts are fudgsicles, sherbet, and frozen low-fat yogurt. The chocolate or carob-covered yogurt bars, however, are not low in fat.

About Cheeses and Cream

Most hard cheeses are high in fat. But cheese merchants are giving us some lower-fat choices these days. Switch to cheeses labeled "part-skim" or to some of the low-fat sliced cheeses, such as Lite-line, Light 'n Lively, and Weight Watchers brand. Mozzarella and jarlsberg are the most common part-skim cheeses. Check the label, though. Some brands of mozzarella are made with whole milk. Sodium-watchers cannot use the low-fat sliced cheeses; like most processed cheeses, these contain large amounts of sodium.

Heavy drinkers of coffee and tea need to think about the creamers added thoughout the day. If skim or low-fat milk is used, there is no problem. But some creamers—half and half, cream, or nondairy whiteners—can quickly raise your fat intake. Use these sparingly; better yet, pick a low-fat replacement.

Help Your Budget and Your Health

Eating more low-fat dairy products will not cost more money. On the contrary, you usually save money when you trim the dairy fat from your diet.

Here are a few examples to think about. These prices were recorded in a Washington, D.C., supermarket in October 1982.

- A half gallon of skim milk costs 89 cents; the same amount of whole milk costs 98 cents.
- Dannon plain low-fat yogurt is priced at 51 cents per cup; Breakstone sour cream costs 87 cents per cup.
- A pound of Breakstone cottage cheese sells for $1.43, while the higher-fat alternative, Fierro ricotta cheese, costs $1.91 per pound.
- The store-brand part-skim mozzarella cheese is priced at $2.85 per pound; store-brand swiss

cheese, made from whole milk, costs $2.99 per pound.

- Top-quality ice cream (Breyer's) sells for $2.59 per half gallon. The top-quality ice milk (Light 'n Lively) runs $2.09 per half gallon. Both are made by the same company.
- A half gallon of store-brand ice cream costs 20 cents more than the same amount of the store-brand ice milk ($1.99 versus $1.79).

There are a few exceptions to this rule. These usually involve newly developed products. Low-fat cheese slices, for instance, are no less expensive than high-fat American cheese. The new reduced-fat cream cheese costs considerably more than the standard cream cheese.

But in general, it is fair to say that eating low-fat dairy products reduces your fat intake, your calorie intake, and your dairy food bill.

Trimming the Meat Fat

Foods in the meat group are a major source of fat in most diets. But contrary to popular belief, you can eat less fat without drastically cutting your meat intake.

Three guidelines are very important:

- Trim as much fat from red meats as possible.
- Favor the leanest cuts of beef, lamb, and pork.
- Replace some of the red meat in your diet with poultry and fish.

There is some fat neatly hidden within the muscle of red meat. It is called marbled fat. But most of the fat is around the outside of the meat and in large, visible chunks within the meat. In other words, much of the fat in meat can be seen and cut away.

A 4-ounce, untrimmed portion of club steak, for instance, contains an incredible 46 grams of fat! Trim the obvious fat from the steak, and the fat count falls to 15 grams. The calorie count drops from an astronomical 515 to 277.

The Best of Beef and Veal

The fat content of a specific cut of meat varies from one piece to another. One round steak might have 7 grams of fat, while another of the same weight might have 10 grams. In general, though, you can count on the following cuts of beef to be reasonably lean:

- rump and round roasts
- round steaks and flank steaks, sometimes called "London broil"
- some sirloin steaks

The following cuts of beef have earned a reputation as fatty:

- rib roast
- porterhouse, T-bone, and club steaks
- beef ribs

Unless labeled "extra lean," hamburger is also rich in fat. Use ground round instead. Ask the butcher to grind a round steak for you if your supermarket doesn't offer ground round.

Veal is usually very lean, except for the veal breast. For the meat-lover willing to pay the price, veal is the perfect beef replacement.

Lean Cuts of Lamb and Pork

Lamb accounts for little of our red meat intake. When you do buy it, though, favor the leg or loin cuts. These are the leanest.

The leanest cut of pork is ham. Fresh ham earns high marks but often is hard to find. Most ham, of course, is cured. Cured meats contain large amounts of salt, as well as the food additive called sodium nitrite. These salt-cured foods are on the "eat less" list of the Committee on Diet, Nutrition, and Cancer. Their cancer-promoting potential will be discussed in the chapter about food additives.

The meat counter does offer some other cuts of pork that have only a moderate fat content. Pork loin and shoulder cuts have more fat than ham but less than fatty cuts such as spareribs.

About Processed Meats

More than two-thirds of the pork produced in the United States ends up as processed meat. The following foods fall under this category:

- bacon and sausages
- hot dogs
- all types of salami
- liverwurst, bologna, and other luncheon meats made from pork

The fat content of these foods is high. And these foods have other strikes against them: a high salt content and the additive sodium nitrite.

There are alternatives to these foods. Some are better than others. Chicken and turkey hot dogs, for example, have less fat than franks made from red meat. But these, too, have a hefty dose of salt, as well as sodium nitrite.

Try to put other fillings inside of sandwiches: lean roast beef, sliced checken, or tuna salad. Not as good but preferable to high-fat fillings are processed poultry products such as turkey breast. Often these items are low in fat but have a generous sprinkling of salt.

Check the label if you are not sure of the fat content. A fat content of 3 to 5 grams per serving is low; above 10 grams per serving is high.

Canadian bacon is preferable to the usual varieties because it has less fat. But all bacon has added salt and is cured with sodium nitrite. If you find bacon irresistible, try Canadian bacon instead. Another good approach is to limit your bacon to two slices; when you eat only small amounts, the fat content is not too unreasonable.

But do consider some alternatives to bacon and sausages. Try cooked potatoes that have been fried in only a small amount of oil. Better yet, fry them with no oil—use a nonstick cooking spray instead.

You can also oven-fry potatoes. Slice cooled, cooked potatoes; season them with one or more spices (garlic, onion, and chili powders are good). Place on a cookie sheet that has been teated with nonstick cooking spray, and bake at 350° until both sides are nicely browned. Turn once during baking.

About Fish and Fowl

In general, fish and poultry are lower in fat than red meat. Also, these foods are almost always lower in saturated fat than red meats. That is why heart experts have been advising us to eat more chicken and fish.

Chicken-lovers should be aware of a few facts:

- White meat chicken (the breast) is the leanest part.
- Dark meat chicken has more fat than white meat, but the fat content is still moderate.
- The skin of all fowl—including duck, goose, and turkey—contains the lion's share of its fat. Part with the skin if you will, or eat only some of it.
- New chicken-raising techniques have caused a sharp increase in the fat content of chicken. But most of the extra fat occurs as "pads" under the skin. These can be removed easily.

Fish Gets First Prize

Fish is the real winner when it comes to fat. Most types have very little fat. Some of the lowest-fat fish are

- abalone
- black sea bass
- cod
- flounder
- haddock
- halibut, Atlantic or Pacific
- pollock
- rockfish
- sole

Even many shellfish contain little fat—despite their reputation for outstanding flavor. This is more evidence that fat and flavor don't always go hand in hand.

Among the low-fat shellfish are such favorites as clams, oysters, crab, lobster, and scallops. Shrimp are also low in fat, but they have a higher count of dietary cholesterol than other shellfish. The role of dietary cholesterol in heart disease is well established. It is still too soon to say whether it plays a role in cancer.

A few fish do bear the label of "fatty." But this means "fatty when compared to other fish," rather than when compared to other foods. The fattier fish include the following:

- anchovies
- herring
- mackerel
- red or chinook salmon
- sablefish
- sardines
- whitefish

These fish have about as much fat as the average cut of red meat.

There is one more category of fish: the canned ones that are often the most reasonably priced. When packed in water, the fat content of chunk light tuna is low. The oil-packed version is rich in fat. If as much oil as possible is drained from the fish, the fat content is moderate.

Albacore tuna presents a problem for fat-watchers. The albacore tuna caught by United States fishermen is not low in fat, but imported albacore is. Check the label in hope of finding what type of albacore is waiting inside.

Pink salmon has a moderate fat content—less than red salmon. Chub salmon also has a moderate fat content. Favor pink and chub over cans labeled "red, King, sockeye, or chinook."

Canned mackerel, herring, and sardines have more fat than tuna or pink salmon. And the oil that is often added makes the fat content higher still. Cut down on these fattier varieties. Or try to find brands that don't contain added oil.

Cooking Tips for Red Meat

Fat matters not only to nutritionists but also to cooks. The fat content of meat, poultry, and fish affects its cooking properties. For good results, you need to know the cooking methods that work best with the leanest meats, poultry, and fish.

Here are some suggestions for getting the most flavor from lean meats:

- Marinate the meat, preferably with little or no oil.
- Cook only to the rare or medium stage, unless you are cooking pork. It should be cooked until well done to prevent trichinosis.
- When cooking in liquid, use low to medium flame.
- Slice meat thin—it will be far more tender.

Some people also like the results when lean meats are cooked in a slow cooker or crock-pot. I prefer a clay pot for cooking lean meats. The results are surprisingly good.

Chicken Cookery

When it comes to cooking chicken, consider the following facts:

- White meat chicken responds best to dry heat. Baking is the best choice.

- Dark meat chicken does well under both dry and moist heat. A recipe that requires cooking the chicken in liquid will taste better if dark meat chicken is used.
- To keep the meat from drying out, don't remove the skin until after cooking.
- When cooking poultry in liquid, skim off any fat that accumulates on the surface.

Needless to say, frying chicken adds to its fat content. Try oven-fried chicken instead (see Unfried Chicken in the recipe section). If you must fry, pan-fry the meat in a small amount of oil. This adds less fat than deep-fat frying.

Fish Cookery

Steaming, baking, and poaching are the best of the traditional methods for cooking fish. A microwave oven is equally as good, and the results are excellent. Broiling is another way to prepare fish without adding fat. For reasons I will discuss later, though, it is probably best not to broil fish all the time.

A low-fat fish can quickly become a high-fat dish if topped with cream sauce or lots of butter. Replace some of the fat often added to fish during cooking with wines. When preparing a white sauce, favor thin sauces; these require less fat. Replace whole milk or cream with skim or low-fat milk.

Like chicken, fish can be oven-fried. Coat it with a seasoned mixture of cornflake crumbs or flour. You can vary the spices and herbs used to make the coating, creating dozens of different dishes. Dip the fish in yogurt or milk first so that the coating mix will adhere.

If frying fish is a must, sauté it in a pan using only

a small amount of margarine, butter, or oil. Fish fried in this way will have less fat than deep-fried fish.

You can lower the fat content of tuna and salmon salads by following these suggestions:

- Buy water-packed fish.
- Use the mayonnaise-type salad dressing (such as Miracle Whip) or "diet mayonnaise" instead of regular mayonnaise; these have only half as much fat.
- Substitute low-fat cottage cheese or yogurt for some of the mayonnaise in tuna or salmon salad.

About High-Cholesterol Foods

Some kinds of meat, poultry, and fish are fairly low in fat, but high in cholesterol. Fat and cholesterol are not the same thing. When it comes to heart disease, however, both saturated fat and cholesterol play a role.

Whether cholesterol in food also plays a role in causing cancer is not known. There is some evidence that a low-cholesterol diet will help to prevent cancer. But the amount of evidence is too small for making judgment.

The best course of action is to keep cholesterol intake, as well as fat intake, at a moderate level. It will help your heart and possibly help prevent other diseases, too.

Three types of food are notably high in cholesterol:

- eggs (actually, the yolk only)
- organ meats
- shrimp

Of these foods, organ meats are by far the highest in cholesterol. Shrimp is only moderately high by comparison.

Most people don't eat organ meats often, but if you do, you should know these facts:

- Of organ meats, brains contain the most cholesterol.
- Kidneys of any animal and chicken liver come in second for cholesterol content.
- Beef liver, sweetbreads, and heart have less than these others but still quite a bit.

If you are a shrimp-lover, rest assured that a shrimp cocktail carries only a moderate cholesterol count. It is when shrimp is eaten in larger amounts—by the cup—that the cholesterol adds up.

How Many Eggs?

In most diets, eggs supply far more cholesterol than organ meats or shrimp. A good rule of thumb is to limit egg intake to three or four a week. This is especially important for people who have high blood cholesterol levels or other risk factors for heart disease: high blood pressure, smoking, diabetes, or obesity.

One easy approach is to use the egg allowance for the usual egg dishes such as scrambled eggs and fried eggs. Then find replacements for the eggs used in casseroles, baking, and other multi-ingredient recipes.

One or more of the following often will successfully replace an egg used in cooking:

- one and a half to two egg whites
- one egg white plus one teaspoon of oil

- one-fourth cup of an egg substitute, preferably one containing no added oil

If you are on a sodium-restricted diet, check with your doctor or dietician before using an egg substitute. None are high in sodium (unless treated with the salt shaker). But these substitutes do have more sodium than eggs.

About Alternatives to Meat

One of the greatest myths about nutrition is the widely held notion that only meat can supply the protein that we need for good health. There is not, and there has never been, any scientific evidence that this is so.

As a matter of fact, there is overwhelming evidence that this idea is purely fiction.

Consider these facts:

- A cup of navy beans has the same protein and calorie count of a hamburger patty.
- A cup of lentils has 2 grams more protein than 2 ounces of cheddar cheese; the lentils have slightly fewer calories.
- Two tablespoons of peanut butter have a little more protein than the cheese or the hamburger.

Few people realize it, but beans, lentils, and nuts have protein that rivals that of meat, poultry, and fish. For this reason, nutritionists put these foods right alongside meats.

With only a few exceptions, the fat content of these "meat alternates" is low. That is why we should use them to replace some of the fatty meats in our diets.

The following members of this group have moderate to high amounts of fat:

- nuts, which are high in fat
- peanut butter, also high in fat
- soybeans, with a moderate fat count
- tofu, another food with a moderate level of fat

Because nuts and nut butters contain mostly unsaturated fat, they belong in our diets if used to replace some of the foods high in saturated fat. By the way, the amount of vegetable oil added to peanut butter is very small. The common commercial brands (Skippy, Jif, Peter Pan) have about the same fat content as "natural" peanut butter.

The Oversold Notion of "Protein Quality"

What about the quality of these plant proteins as compared to animal proteins? That is the second part of the protein myth.

Though animal proteins do have higher-quality protein than most vegetable foods, most adults simply do not need the extra protein that meat provides.

Vegetarians prove this point beautifully. Most vegetarians eat dairy products and eggs, which provide more than enough protein. But even adult vegetarians who eat no animal products at all have been found to eat about twice the minimum requirement of each protein that humans need.

Some people do have to take special care if eating diets containing no animal protein. In this category are

- preschool children
- pregnant and nursing women

- people eating large amounts of sugars and fats and oils
- people recovering from severe infections or other kinds of trauma

The record shows that vegetable protein can meet the protein needs of people in these situations. But care and planning are required. Grains and legumes should be combined to provide high-quality protein, and soy foods should be eaten regularly.

Fruits and Vegetables

By now, you have heard me rave about fruits and vegetables at least ten times. You don't have to look up the fat content of each one. With only three exceptions, all are very low in fat.

The exceptions are

- olives
- avocados
- coconut

The first exception rarely matters for most people. A single olive has only half a gram of fat. Most people eat only one or two at a time—on a salad or as a garnish. Eaten in this way, the fat content is negligible. (Sodium-watchers, though, should leave olives on the plate.)

Eat the whole jar of olives, and the story changes. Then the fat starts to add up.

Coconut and avocado contain a great deal of fat. Eat them in small amounts.

The Misunderstood Starches

The most underrated foods in our diet are the starches. Foods such as bread, pasta, rice, and cereal deserve high marks. Instead, they have been put down as fattening and non-nutritious.

In the history of nutrition, there never has been a worse misconception. We should be eating more of these starches. Yet many people avoid them.

Most foods rich in starch have a lot going for them. Foods in this group usually have the following good points:

- a moderate calorie count
- B-vitamins
- significant amounts of protein
- iron and other minerals
- fiber and high levels of some minerals unless refined.

And the most important plus of all: *very little fat.*

Occasionally, food companies take low-fat ingredients, such as flour or oats, and douse them in fat. The only cereal with significant amounts of added fat is granola. Its fat content is moderate; add whole milk and the fat content jumps.

Croissants, sometimes called crescent rolls, are quite high in fat. Very flaky biscuits also may be rich in fat. But other rolls contain at most moderate levels of fat. Virtually all loaf breads are low in fat.

At the table, try not to overdo the margarine, butter, or cream cheese. It is the fat added to starchy foods, not the foods themselves, that makes them fattening.

Desserts Can Be Low in Fat, Too!

If you are tired of beig told to eat fruit for dessert, read on. Of course, fruit is an ideal dessert: low in fat and often rich in certain vitamins. But most people want more variety than fruits provide. On a low-fat diet, there *are* more options than fruit alone.

The following desserts are low in fat:

- angel food cake (no fat at all!)
- some gingerbread recipes
- fig bars
- raisin-fruit biscuits
- gingersnaps
- some brands of ice milk
- fudgsicles
- sherbet
- pretzels
- hard candy

In general, cakes have less fat than cookies. Chocolate cakes and pound cakes are often higher in fat than other varieties. Many prepared cakes and cake mixes now carry nutrition information; try to choose products that supply no more than 7 grams of fat per serving.

Fruit fillings for pies are usually low in fat. The crust is the troublemaker—it is almost always rich in fat. The best thing that a pie-lover can do is to choose one-crust pies over two-crust pies. When possible, use the oat pie crust given in the recipe section. It has a reasonable fat content.

Commercial pudding mixes contain only small amounts of fat. If prepared with low-fat or skim milk, these products can be used on a low-fat diet.

If you make your own cakes, pies, and puddings, you can often have desserts that are lower in sodium, sugar, and fat than commercial products. But if you cannot make your own, following these guidelines will help you keep your fat intake at a moderate level.

The Fats and Oils Story

A hundred years ago, shoppers had few fats to choose from. Usually, only butter and lard were available to consumers.

Today, there are enough fats and oils on the market to confuse anyone. But all of them fall into one of three categories:

• table fats (butter and margarines)
• cooking and salad oils
• shortenings

To make things simpler, remember just one thing. All of these items are high in fat. In fact, the fat content of shortenings and oils is virtually identical. Butter and margarine have slightly less fat because these spreads contain a small amount of water that shortenings and oils lack.

The Different Types of Fat

The only important difference between the many fats has to do with what nutritionists call "type of fat." Some of the fat in food is saturated, while other fats are monounsaturated or polyunsaturated. In the next section, we will look closely at the type of fat in food. The saturated type of fat promotes heart disease, but others don't seem to do so.

But when it comes to cancer prevention, all fats are on equal footing. Scientists believe that eating less of any type of fat will help prevent cancers of the breast, colon, and prostate gland. They have not concluded that any one type of fat has more effect on cancer than another.

This makes the message about fat and cancer much simpler than advice on preventing heart disease.

You need only to keep three guidelines in mind concerning the fats and oils in your diet:

- Add no more than one pat of margarine to each serving of bread, pasta, or vegetables.
- Limit fats and oils used in cooking to no more than two tablespoons per four servings (three tablespoons for six servings).
- Experiment with reduced-fat salad dressings, margarines, and cream cheese; try jams, jellies, and other condiments to replace some or all of the fat added to food.

Saturated or Unsaturated?

For those who are interested in preventing both heart disease and cancer, I would like to offer some facts about the type of fat in food.

Preventing heart disease means eating less saturated fat, for saturated fat raises the blood cholesterol level. High blood cholesterol is one of the three major factors that determine your risk of heart disease.

The polyunsaturated fats help to lower the blood cholesterol. But these fats don't lower blood cholesterol as efficiently as saturated fats raise it. Eating less saturated fat is the most important thing to do.

All foods contain some of each type of fat. That makes life too complicated, though, because it means that everything is partially saturated, partially mono-unsaturated, and partially polyunsaturated. Nutritionists have simplified things, calling a fat saturated or unsaturated based on the amount of each fat that the food contains.

The following kinds of fat have enough saturated fat to be simply called saturated:

- beef, pork, or lamb fats
- milkfat and butter
- coconut and palm oils
- some industrial shortenings

Industrial shortenings are those used by food companies to make processed foods. Supermarkets do not sell these shortenings, but we encounter them in a wide range of ready-made products. Most vegetable oils and some margarines fall into the polyunsaturated category. There are many to choose from. They include

- corn oil
- safflower oil
- sesame seed oil
- soybean oil
- sunflower oil
- some margarines, most likely those in tubs

Olive oil, peanut oil, many margarines, and some industrial shortenings are monounsaturated. The monounsaturated fats have little or no effect on the blood cholesterol level.

Chicken and fish fats are less saturated than the fat of red meats. For this reason, nutritionists and heart experts recommend eating more fish and fowl.

Fat and Calories

We will probably learn a lot about weight control between now and the year 2000. I am willing to bet, though, that the bottom line on reducing diets will be the same then as it is now. *The best way to diet is to eat less fat.*

The explanation is nothing that a first-grader couldn't understand. Fat has more calories than anything else in food.

- Protein has four calories per gram.
- Carbohydrate has four calories per gram.
- Alcohol has seven calories per gram.
- Fat has *nine* calories per gram.

Little wonder that obesity is common in nations that have high-fat diets. (If you are wondering what a gram of fat looks like, it measures a little less than a quarter of a teaspoon.)

If you follow the recommendations in this chapter, you will almost certainly reduce your calorie intake. It is just another reason, among many, to eat less fat.

The Weight Watchers diet, by the way, contains 30 percent of calories from fat, the same figure recommended by the Committee on Diet, Nutrition, and Cancer.

Can Eating Less Fat Be Harmful?

Most nutritionists would laugh if asked this question. For decades, nutritionists have known that the body needs only about 10 percent of its calories from fat. The American diet averages four times that.

The one warning about cutting back on fat pertains only to infants. Children under one year of age should not be fed a low-fat diet unless ordered by a doctor. The reason is simple: during the first year of life, many infants need the extra calories that fat provides.

This concern about infants aside, scientists stress that there is no known harm to cutting back on fat to the level recommended by the Committee on Diet, Nutrition, and Cancer. Public health experts cannot help but notice that Japanese life expectancy is among the highest in the world. Yet fat intake in Japan is far lower than in other industrialized nations.

I have been watching my fat intake ever since I was a graduate student. I hope I have convinced you to do the same.

9

Alcohol

Focus on this chapter if you smoke cigarettes.

It is no secret that too much alcohol causes all kinds of trouble: traffic accidents; family problems; liver disease; even nutrient deficiencies. And now, it is almost certain that cancer will be added to the list of woes.

But the research linking alcohol to cancer doesn't have scientists advocating a return to Prohibition. They are calling for a sensible, moderate approach.

It is *excessive drinking* that concerns the cancer experts. Overconsumption of alcohol has been linked to cancers of the stomach, colon, and rectum.

Research also shows that heavy drinking combined with smoking greatly magnifies the chance of developing other forms of cancer. Cancer of the mouth, throat, and esophagus is often the result of mixing too much alcohol with cigarette smoking.

I write this chapter, by the way, from the perspective of a near-teetotaler. I never have been much of a drinker.

I feel, however, than an objective discussion about alcohol should cover its role in heart disease as well as in cancer. The latest findings in heart disease show that *modest* drinking reduces a man's chances of having a heart attack. Heart disease, of course, is far more common than the cancers linked to alcohol.

So, in my opinion, talking about alcohol means looking at the whole picture. Here it is.

The Recommendation and How to Meet It.

"Drink alcohol only in moderation." That's the word from both the National Cancer Institute and the Committee on Diet, Nutrition, and Cancer.

Dr. Arthur Upton, the former director of the National Cancer Institute, gave his group's advice at a Senate hearing in 1979. The senators immediately wanted to know what he meant by the term "moderation."

It was a good question. Too often, it goes unanswered. When it does, we are at a loss to know what to do.

Upton defined "moderate drinking" as fewer than three drinks per day. If pressed for an answer, most health experts would probably agree that one to two drinks per day qualifies as a moderate intake.

I am not going to pretend that there is a substitute for alcoholic beverages that tastes similar to the real thing. Cutting down on alcohol basically means having fewer drinks.

An Important Definition

In nutrition, the word "alcohol" has two meanings. The term is often used loosely when referring to any of the various beverages that contain alcohol. It is not unusual to hear beer, wine, or mixed drinks described simply as "alcohol."

Strictly speaking, though, none of these beverages are purely alcohol. They contain water, and some contain carbohydrates. In other words, alcohol is only one of the components in wine, beer, and mixed drinks.

In this book, the word "alcohol" is used in the strict sense. It applies only to the portion of a drink that is actually alcohol. Presumably, it is only the alcohol portion of these beverages that accounts for their ill effects.

Some Alternatives

Having fewer drinks is the best way to cut down on your alcohol intake, and for many people it's the only way. But in some cases, there are other ways to make modest changes in your alcohol intake.

If you do the mixing yourself, you can reduce the alcohol content of mixed drinks by using less alcohol and more of the nonalcoholic ingredients. The recipe section includes some wine punches that use fruit juice to lower the alcohol content.

In bars and restaurants, bartenders are almost always willing to comply with a request for a weaker drink.

Finally, the alcohol content can vary among the different kinds of drinks. Choosing the beers, wines, and mixed drinks that are lowest in alcohol content can make a difference in the alcohol and *calorie* content of your diet. Read on to learn how.

Rating the Drinks

The alcohol content of wines and spirits is listed on the label. It lets you compare among different brands of the same beverage.

What it doesn't let you do is compare wine to

spirits. Why not? Because we drink them in such different amounts. The standard serving of wine is 4 ounces, while the typical mixed drink has 1½ ounces (one jigger) of gin, vodka, rum, or whiskey.

Needless to say, it is also impossible to compare wines to beer, or beers to mixed drinks, because only some beer cans show the alcohol content.

But with the help of my calculator and some food composition tables, I have been able to make some estimates.

Here is how drinks compare:

- A 12-ounce can or bottle of regular beer has about 13 grams of alcohol.
- A 12-ounce can or bottle of "lite" beer contains about 10 grams of alcohol—about 25 percent less than regular beer.
- A 4-ounce glass of table wine has about 11 grams of alcohol. (Four ounces is about half a cup.)
- A mixed drink made with one jigger of 80 proof whiskey, vodka, gin, or rum has about 14 grams of alcohol.

Admittedly, the differences listed above are small. But there is a catch.

My figures are based on typical beers, wines, and mixed drinks. The alcohol content of one winery's chablis can be different from another's. The law sets a limit on the alcohol content of table wines but permits a sizable range in alcohol content.

The same holds true for beers and distilled spirits (whiskey, rum, gin, and vodka). The alcohol content of both "lite" and regular beers varies from one brewery to another. In some cases, the differences are large.

In upcoming sections, we'll take a closer look at each type of alcohol.

A Success Story: Nitrosamines in Beer

A few years ago, reporter Roberta Baskin of Chicago's WLS-TV shook up her viewers with some startling revelations.

Tests done at her station's request showed significant levels of nitrosamines in most of the common brands of beer. Nitrosamines, of course, are the powerful cancer-causing agent suspected in cancers of the stomach and esophagus.

Bacon has always been in the spotlight as the most common source of nitrosamines in food. But Baskin calculated that Americans were getting far more nitrosamines from beer because we consume far more beer than bacon.

Scientists and brewers quickly untangled the mystery. The source of the nitrosamines was the malt used in making beer. When malt was dried in the usual way, nitrosamines developed.

The Food and Drug Administration confirmed that a problem existed and set limits on the nitrosamine content of beer and malt. Brewers have apparently had little trouble complying with the new rules. They have switched to malt made by a different process.

Whether these nitrosamines in beer account for the findings linking heavy beer drinking to cancers of the colon and rectum is anybody's guess. But there is little doubt that today's beers have far lower nitrosamine levels than in the past.

A Closer Look at Beer

If you are a beer-drinker, you may be interested in a survey taken by the Center for Science in the Public Interest, where I formerly worked.

The center's survey showed that alcohol content varies among different brands of beer. Among regular beers, it ranges from 3.2 percent (by volume) to 5 percent by volume. That means that some beers have about 50 percent more alcohol than others!

The regular beers having the lowest alcohol content by volume were

- Stroh Bohemian (3.2 percent)
- Schmidt Low-Alcohol (3.2 percent)
- Budweiser Low-Alcohol (3.9 percent)
- Busch Bavarian Low-Alcohol (3.9 percent)

Here is the other side of the story. The regular beers having the highest alcohol content were

- Black Horse Ale (5.0 percent)
- Busch Bavarian (4.9 percent)
- Budweiser (4.9 percent)
- Michelob (4.9 percent)

Rheingold, Meister Brau Premium, Knickerbocker, Buck-eye, and Heidelberg reported an alcohol content of 4.6 percent. The USDA food composition tables that list the calorie and nutrient values of food assume that beer has this level of alcohol.

As I noted earlier, lite beers have less alcohol than regular beers. In the Center for Science in the Public Interest survey, three brands of lite beer stood out.

These three have an alcohol content of less than 3 percent by volume. They are

- Pabst Extra Light (2.4 percent)
- Pearl Light (2.8 percent)
- Burgie! Light Golden (2.9 percent)

The lite beers with highest alcohol content were Gablinger's Extra Light and Meister Brau Lite, with 4.5 percent and 4.6 percent alcohol respectively.

The Word on Table Wines

Table wines, as a group, have less alcohol than dessert wines. In its food tables, the USDA classifies the following as table wines.

- barbera
- burgundy
- cabernet
- chablis
- champagne
- chianti
- claret
- Rhine wine
- rose
- sauterne

By the way, red table wines do not have a notably different alcohol or calorie count from white table wines.

Among table wines, the dry varieties often have a little more alcohol than the sweeter ones. A sweeter wine probably has more of the sugar that occurs naturally in grapes. In drier wines, the sugar has turned to alcohol.

Incidentally, the new "lite" table wines have even less alcohol than the regular table wines. They have fewer calories, too.

Dessert Wines Differ

Dessert wines contain more alcohol than table wines. This difference can be small or large, depending on the winery. Food composition tables compiled by the USDA show that the average dessert wine has 50 percent more alcohol than the average table wine.

If you drink dessert wines in much smaller amounts than table wine, the difference probably is not important. But if you drink them in similar amounts, the dessert wine will give you more alcohol.

Dessert wines also have a slightly higher carbohydrate count than table wines. Added to the higher alcohol content, this makes for quite a few more calories, as we'll see in an upcoming section.

The USDA includes the following varieties in its list of dessert wines:

- apple and muscatel
- port and tokay
- sherries and vermouths
- "aperitif" wines

The Cocktail Connection

Cocktails usually contain gin, rum, vodka, or whiskey. The "whiskey" category includes a wide range of products: rye, corn, and blended whiskies, as well as bourbon and scotch. Collectively, these products are known as distilled spirits.

No doubt you know that the proof of distilled

spirits represents their alcohol content. These distilled spirits, as well as brandy, are typically 80 proof. As mentioned earlier, a drink made with a jigger of 80 proof spirits has only a little more alcohol than a glass of wine or a can of beer.

But some brands are greater than 80 proof. And some are less.

The difference in alcohol content between 80 proof and 86 or 90 proof is small. A jigger of 90 proof liquor, for instance, has about 2 more grams of alcohol than 80 proof. That is not much. But the alcohol content of 100 proof spirits goes higher still. After a few drinks made with 100 proof instead of 80 proof, the extra alcohol starts to add up.

Here are some examples of whiskey that are 100 proof or more. All are based on a survey taken in 1982.

- J. W. Dant, I. W. Harper, and Old Grand Dad bond bourbon (100 proof)
- Old Grand Dad Special Selection straight bourbon (114 proof) and Wild Turkey straight bourbon (101 proof)
- Four Queens blended whiskey (101 proof) and Black Bull scotch whiskey (100 proof)

Vodka, Gin, and Rum

A number of vodkas are 100 proof, though there are plenty of 80 proof vodkas. Companies that make 100 proof vodka also make 80 proof vodka. You have to check the label to know whether you have chosen the version with the higher alcohol count.

The following nine companies make both 80 and 100 proof vodkas:

- Gilbey's
- Gordon's
- Jacquin's Royale
- Kasser's Kavkaski
- Nikolai
- Old Mr. Boston
- Ostrova
- Smirnoff
- Stolichnaya (imported from the USSR)

Last but not least are the rums and gins. I found no gins in my survey that are 100 proof or more. But I did find two brands of rum with a whopping 151 proof: Barcardi 151 and Ronrico 151.

Using more than one jigger of gin, rum, vodka, or whiskey in a drink will obviously hike the alcohol content. Drinks that are combinations of two kinds of alcohol—such as martinis and manhattans—will have slightly more alcohol than drinks that mix a jigger of liquor with fruit juices or sodas.

Specialty Liquors

Some distilled spirits don't fall under the category of whiskey, vodka, rum, or gin. They are known as specialties or cordials.

Most products in this category are lower than 80 proof. But before I list them, here are a few that are 100 proof:

- Southern Comfort
- Old Southern
- Yukon Jack Liqueur

The proof of other cordials and specialties varies widely. Some are as low as 32 proof, while others, such as Grand Marnier, are the standard 80 proof.

If you drink cordials in the same amount that you would use whiskey, gin, and the like, you can cut down on your alcohol intake by using cordials having a low proof. But if you drink twice as much of a cordial, substituting it for whiskey does not reduce your alcohol intake.

You will need to check the label of different brands to be sure of the alcohol content. *In general,* though, the following cordials have a proof of 60 or less:

- anisette and amaretto
- coffee liqueur and cream liqueur
- creme de menthe, creme de cacao, and creme de almond, banana, or strawberry
- triple sec and peppermint schnapps

The Heart's Desire?

At the beginning of this chapter, I mentioned that research links *moderate* alcohol consumption to a lower risk of heart disease.

Most heart attacks result from fatty deposits that clog and harden the arteries that supply the heart with blood. The most common type of cholesterol in the blood, LDL-cholesterol, is the guilty party. It promotes this clogging process.

Foods rich in saturated fat and cholesterol raise the amount of LDL-cholesterol in the blood. This high cholesterol level, in turn, encourages the clogging of the arteries.

As far as we know, alcohol does not affect the level of LDL-cholesterol. What it does seem to affect is the amount of another component of blood. This component is called HDL-cholesterol.

The HDL-cholesterol is linked to lower risk of heart disease. You might say that its effects are the opposite of those of LDL-cholesterol. Rather than promote the clogging process, it apparently helps to slow it down.

Research shows that men who regularly drink small amounts of alcohol have higher levels of HDL-cholesterol than do nondrinkers. Whether this is also true for women is unknown. Few heart studies have been done with women.

Other factors linked to a healthy level of HDL-cholesterol are exercise, normal weight, and non-smoking.

Drinking a great deal on the weekend but almost none during the week does not qualify as moderate drinking. And heavy drinkers do not do well at all when it comes to heart disease. They have a greater than average risk.

Although a number of studies show similar results regarding moderate drinking and heart disease, we have yet to learn how drinking affects total life expectancy. We cannot interpret the research on heart disease to mean that moderate drinkers live longer than nondrinkers. We do not know that this is so.

But more Americans die of heart attacks than cancers (or other diseases) linked to alcohol. For this reason, I am not ready to say that moderate drinkers should not drink at all.

Neither, it seems, is the Committee on Diet, Nutrition, and Cancer. Its advice, again, is to drink alcohol only in moderation.

Remember the Calories

When you do enjoy an alcoholic beverage, remember that it is not a diet drink. The calories in these drinks add up—quickly.

Here are a few numbers that speak for themselves:

- A regular beer (12-ounce bottle or can) averages about 150 calories.
- "Lite" beers average about 100 calories per 12 ounces—a respectable savings.
- A 4-ounce glass of table wine has about 80 to 100 calories.
- A 4-ounce glass of dessert wine has anywhere from 130 to 260 calories.

The lower-calorie choices are obvious. As for distilled spirits, here are the USDA's values for whiskey, gin, rum, and vodka:

- 80 proof (1 jigger):   95 calories
- 86 proof (1 jigger): 105 calories
- 90 proof (1 jigger): 110 calories
- 100 proof (1 jigger): 124 calories

Of course, you add other ingredients to that jigger: fruit juice, vermouth, and soda, to name a few. Using recipes in *Mr. Boston Deluxe Official Bartender's Guide*, the Center for Science in the Public Interest calculated the calorie count of some popular mixed drinks. For making the calculations, 86 proof liquor was used.

The results looked like this:

- bloody mary: 125 calories
- martini: 130 calories
- manhattan: 140 calories
- whiskey sour or old-fashioned: 160 calories
- gin and tonic: 195 calories
- rum and coke: 210 calories
- screwdriver: 230 calories

I can often be heard saying that eating less fat is the best way to lose weight. But these numbers make clear that drinking less alcohol comes in a close second.

10
Food Additives

Two decades ago, few of us gave much thought to food additives. But in 1969, some startling findings confronted us. A respected scientist warned that a food additive in baby food could cause brain damage in infant mice.

Baby food manufacturers soon removed that additive, monosodium glutamate (MSG), from their products. The shock waves lingered, nonetheless. Consumers and scientists alike became wary about food additives. The greatest fear, of course, was that food additives might cause cancer.

Like other nutrition-minded consumers, I, too, was suspicious of food additives. Unlike some, I did not dismiss all additives as guilty. But if you had asked me what aspect of food might influence cancer, food additives would have been my reply.

After years of studying the subject of nutrition and cancer, I have changed my mind. I no longer think it likely that food additives are a *major* cause of cancer in the United States.

Why the change of heart? First, because rates of most cancers in the United States have not fluctuated much during the last thirty years, despite an enormous increase in the use of food additives. Also, countries such as Japan use food additives yet their cancer patterns bear little resemblance to ours.

Most important, in my mind, though, are the results of studies on animals. In the case of many food additives, laboratory testing has shown little or no reason to fear that these compounds cause cancer.

That is not to say that all additives are 100 percent safe. A few still look suspicious, not only to me, but to others in my field. Among those still concerned about certain additives are the Committee on Diet, Nutrition, and Cancer; the National Cancer Institute; the Food and Drug Administration; and even some food companies.

Nitrite: Still A Prime Suspect

The Committee on Diet, Nutrition, and Cancer made very few recommendations pertaining to food additives. But it did give advice about foods containing the additive sodium nitrite.

"Eat very little salt-cured, salt-pickled and smoked foods," said the panel.

Evidence from around the world convinced the scientists that these cured foods almost certainly play a role in causing cancers of the stomach and esophagus. In fact, scientists believe that diets rich in cured and pickled foods may be a major factor in causing these two forms of cancer. These diseases are common in countries where people often eat cured and pickled foods.

It is no secret why these foods might be able to cause cancer. Nitrite is often used in the curing process. If it remained nitrite in our bodies, there might not be a problem. But, unfortunately, it can be changed into a cancer-causing chemical.

The problem apparently begins when the nitrite combines with substances called amines. This can happen during cooking or in the body. When it does, the notorious substances called nitrosamines can form.

Scientists know that these nitrosamines can cause cancer in dozens of different kinds of animals. Some of the nitrosamines are so powerful that even tiny amounts can cause cancer in test animals.

Meeting the Recommendation

Certain foods are almost always salt-cured. The Committee on Diet, Nutrition, and Cancer has urged us to eat "very little" of them.

Another committee of the National Academy of Sciences, convened solely to study the nitrite problem, also concluded that our exposure to nitrite should be lowered.

These are the salt-cured foods that almost always contain sodium nitrite:

- sausages and bacon
- hot dogs, bologna, liverwurst, and salami
- smoked chicken and turkey products
- smoked fish (lox, kippered salmon, smoked salmon)

If you are in doubt about whether a food is salt-cured, read the label closely. The words *sodium nitrite* and *salt* among the ingredients signal a food that is salt-cured.

The committee scientists also advised us to eat few pickled vegetables. Though sodium nitrite is not used in pickling, scientists believe that these foods contain compounds related to nitrosamines. Researchers have found high rates of esophageal cancer in parts of the world where people eat lots of pickled vegetables.

There Are Alternatives!

It can be Sunday without sausage or bacon on the table. Home fries or hash-brown potatoes, if fried in only small amounts of oil, are also good.

Those who cannot part with bacon can find a nitrite-free version in many health food stores and in some supermarkets. Nitrite-free bacon has been smoked but not with nitrite. It is not known if the smoking process poses a risk even when nitrite is not used. Regardless, nitrite-free meats should pose *less* of a risk than those cured with nitrite.

Imitation bacon strips, made from soybeans, are another alternative to bacon. Similarly, there are imitation soy sausage links and patties. These products can be found in the supermarket freezer case.

These soy products contain no nitrite and are not smoked. Their total fat content is high, but the fat is unsaturated.

That is the up side. On the down side, some people find that these don't taste quite like bacon or sausage. More important, the sodium content is extremely high. Those watching their sodium intake should avoid these products.

For taste, imitation bacon bits (such as "BacOs") sometimes get higher marks than the soy bacon strips and sausages. These imitation bits work very well in salads, eggs, and egg dishes such as quiche.

The imitation bacon bits contain less fat than bacon. Again the salt content is very high, but no nitrites are used. Most of the fat is unsaturated, so those on cholesterol-lowering diets can use this product.

Healthier Sandwiches

Obviously, some of the most common salt-cured foods often appear between slices of bread or rolls: hot dogs, salami, liverwurst, bologna, and other luncheon meats.

The alternatives are obvious: lean roast beef, sliced chicken or turkey, tuna, salmon, or peanut butter.

Nitrite-free hot dogs can be found in many health food stores. Those who enjoy cooking can also make their own hot dogs; no nitrite is needed.

The alternative to pickled vegetables, of course, is the vegetable in its fresh state.

Spice Tips

A few spices can help imitate the flavor that we associate with cured meats. Hickory-smoked salt and liquid smoke add somewhat similar flavor to meats.

Recently, scientists studied these flavorings and concluded that they appear to be safe. But the scientists did point to some unanswered questions and asked that additional testing be done. Until more results are available, it is probably fair to say that these flavorings seem safer than sodium nitrite.

Oregano, sage, and fennel can also be used to add a pungent taste to meats.

"Take with Vitamin C"

If none of these suggestions help, there is one last resort: vitamin C. I already have told you that this familiar vitamin can block the reaction that turns nitrites into cancer-causing nitrosamines.

If you cannot resist salt-cured foods, do yourself a favor and eat a food rich in vitamin C at the same time. Here are some easy ways to do this:

- Drink orange, grapefruit, or tomato juice whenever you eat cured meats.
- Have fruit drinks enriched with vitamin C (for instance, cranberry juice cocktail); these will provide vitamin C but are not as nutritious as citrus or tomato juice.
- Add sliced green pepper or tomato to your sandwich.
- Eat a salad with the meal.
- Enjoy a fruit rich in vitamin C for dessert such as watermelon, cantaloupe, or strawberries.

You may notice that many cured meats list vitamin C as an ingredient. Meat packers use it to stabilize the color and flavor of cured meats. It can serve our health at the same time by helping to block formation of nitrosamines.

The amount of vitamin C added to processed meats is fairly small: less than 10 milligrams per average serving. It is not known whether this is enough to provide strong protection against nitrosamines.

For this reason, it is probably wise to eat fruits or vegetables rich in vitamin C when having cured meats.

The recipe section of this book includes the following dishes in which cured meats are combined with foods rich in vitamin C.

- Orange-Raisin Ham Rolls
- Luncheon Stuffed Peppers

- Ham Sandwich with Vitamin C
- Easy and Elegant Orange Ham

I offer these recipes not with the recommendation that you eat these foods but as a compromise. I recognize that some people are especially fond of cured meats. These recipes are for them.

Rating the Salt-Cured Foods

More than two dozen salt-cured foods can be found in the average supermarket. The Committee on Diet, Nutrition, and Cancer gives them all the "eat rarely" label.

It is not that I disagree. I would simply like to point out that some of these foods are better than others. This way, those who relish cured foods can choose the lesser of evils.

Here is my pecking order for cured meats:

- best of the lot: smoked turkey breast or turkey ham
- second best: well-trimmed lean ham or smoked fish
- third place: poultry luncheon meats other than turkey breast or ham; Canadian bacon
- fourth place: beef or pork hot dogs labeled as reduced in fat
- last: traditional beef and pork sausages, luncheon meats, bacon

As you probably have guessed, my rating system is based on the amount of fat and saturated fat in these foods. Turkey breast and turkey ham are lowest in total fat. Lean, trimmed ham (from pork) has moderate amounts of fat and saturated fat.

Smoked fish contains little saturated fat, though it usually does have a higher fat content than most fish.

The products in third place have a moderate amount of saturated fat. Those in fourth place are high in both fat and saturated fat but slightly less so than the foods in last place.

The Rainbow of Artificial Colors

Here is a rule of thumb on the subject of food additives: *"A simple, general rule about additives is to avoid sodium nitrite and artificial coloring."*

Those words come from *Chemical Cuisine,* a poster designed by my former co-workers at the Center for Science in the Public Interest.

You already know how to avoid sodium nitrite. Avoiding artificial colors is not difficult either. The reason for avoiding these artificial colors is simple. When compared to other additives, these colors have fared most poorly in safety tests.

There are many artificial colors. Yet most of them are closely related. Most colors are coal-tar dyes. Originally, these compounds came from coal tar. Today, scientists can make them synthetically.

It has been more than half a century since coal tar first showed cancer-causing potential in laboratory studies.

Which Foods Have Artificial Colors?

These artificial colors probably do not account for a major portion of cancer cases. Yet it does make sense to avoid them when possible.

Whether one food color is worse than the others is

not really known. As of now, though, a color called Red No. 40 has been the greatest cause for concern. The following foods often contain this dye:

- artificially colored gelatin desserts
- baked goods
- carbonated drinks
- candy

Some processed foods that are red or orange in appearance do not contain Red No. 40. Many cheeses, for instance, obviously have been colored orange. Cheese-makers use anatto, a dye that occurs naturally in the seeds of the anatto plant. There has never been any question about its safety.

Likewise, orange processors do not use Red No. 40 to color the skin of oranges. A dye called Citrus Red No. 2 is used for this purpose. This dye, too, has shown cancer-causing potential in some studies.

Orange-lovers can rest assured that the pulp of the orange does not absorb the dye. You eat the dye only if you eat the peel. Since most people eat the peel only rarely, this should not be a major cause for concern.

One dye that does seem to be safe is Yellow No. 6. It can cause allergic reactions in a few people. But it does not seem to be cancer-causing.

My former colleagues at the Center for Science in the Public Interest felt that other food colorings such as blue and green have not been tested adequately. Until these colors are proved safe, it is probably best to avoid them when possible.

The Sweeteners Story

Low-calorie sweeteners have been around for decades. No doubt they are here to stay.

The following low-calorie sweeteners are in use today:

- saccharine
- aspartame
- sorbitol
- mannitol

Some of these may be safer than others.

The safety of saccharin has been heavily debated in recent years. There is little question that it can cause cancer in laboratory animals when fed in large doses.

Whether these findings are important to humans is a matter of opinion among scientists. Regular use of saccharine may pose a significant risk. But the risk is probably not great; some studies have not found higher rates of cancer among heavy users of saccharin.

Aspartame, saccharin's new competitor, is probably a safer choice. It first became available in 1982 under the brand name Equal.

During digestion, aspartame breaks down into two substances that our bodies encounter every day. Both of these breakdown compounds are found in ordinary protein foods.

Though there have been reports that aspartame can cause cancer in animals, the Food and Drug Administration has concluded otherwise. After reviewing all of the studies, the Food and Drug Administration has concluded that aspartame is safe and does not cause cancer.

Foods sweetened with aspartame will no doubt become more and more common in future years. Aspartame can replace sugar in coffee or tea and be used to sweeten fruits and other foods. It cannot replace sugar used in baking. In cakes and cookies, for instance, sugar contributes to the bulk and texture of the dough.

Another sweetener, mannitol, provides more calories than aspartame or saccharin, but it has only half as many calories as sugar. It is used in a few sugarless products, including chewing gum. On the basis of research now available, there seems little doubt about its safety.

A related substance, sorbitol, is also used in dietetic foods. Occasionally it causes intestinal pain and diarrhea in people who eat large amounts of it. Otherwise, however, sorbitol is considered quite safe. It occurs naturally in fruit and berries.

An Intensive Study of Food Additive Safety

I will not have many more words of caution about food additives. Other than the ones already mentioned, only a few remain suspect in the search for cancer-causing chemicals.

Recently, a major study of food additive safety was completed for the Food and Drug Administration. Years ago, the agency had compiled a list of food ingredients that were assumed to be safe. These substances were "Generally Recognized as Safe (GRAS)."

For more than a decade, virtually no one questioned the safety of using these additives in food. During the 1970s, the Food and Drug Administration decided to reevaluate its list. The agency wanted the safety of each substance to be thoroughly reviewed.

The Food and Drug Administration arranged for an independent group of scientists to evaluate the safety of substances on the GRAS list. The panel was organized by the Federation of American Societies for Experimental Biology (FASEB), a professional society of scientists.

Each Additive Was Rated

The FASEB panel of scientists classified each additive in one of the following categories:

- Class 1: safe at current levels of consumption and at levels that might be expected in the future
- Class 2: safe at current levels, but safety at higher levels is uncertain
- Class 3: appears safe as currently used, but uncertainties exist; better testing is needed
- Class 4: appears harmful at levels now in use; use of the substance should be regulated
- Class 5: no evaluation possible because of a shortage of safety tests with the substance

Most of the additives studied by the FASEB scientists were categorized as Class 1 or Class 2. We will be looking at the most important additives of each category throughout the rest of this chapter. The full results of the FASEB study can be obtained from the Food and Drug Administration; see the Appendix for details.

Obviously, many of the substances added to food did pass the safety test. One reason why is that many common additives are naturally occurring substances.

Some Additives Are Nature's Own

Opponents of food additives sometimes give the chemists a little too much credit. They accuse food technologists of inventing thousands of foreign substances to add to our food.

Often, though, the chemists have not been that creative. They have simply copied Mother Nature's own designs. *Many of the food additives in use are substances that occur naturally in food.*

It may seem strange to classify such substances as additives. But by definition, a naturally occurring substance can in fact be an additive.

A natural substance becomes an additive whenever it is used in a food in which it is not naturally found. Vitamin C, for instance, occurs naturally in oranges. It is not an additive in oranges or in orange juice. On the other hand, vitamin C does not occur naturally in meat. Meat packers who use vitamin C in their products must list it on the label as an additive.

Natural Additives with Exotic Names

Many additives have exotic names that inspire more fear than the words "vitamin C." But the fact is that many naturally occurring substances have been given exotic-sounding names.

Here is my favorite example. Food chemists refer to fats in food as triglycerides. A fat such as butter is composed mostly of triglycerides. Butter also contains two related substances known as monoglycerides and diglycerides. These mono- and diglycerides, of course, occur naturally in butter. Therefore, you will not find them listed on the label.

Margarine, however, does not occur in nature. For this reason, all of its ingredients are listed on the label. Yet some of its strange-sounding ingredients, such as mono- and diglycerides, are nothing more than the natural constituents of butter and other fats.

Some Anti-Cancer Additives

Another common additive not only occurs naturally but may have anti-cancer potential. You have read about it already: carotene. Margarine manufacturers, for example, use carotene for several reasons. One is to give a yellow color.

Carotene is also added to margarine so that it provides as much vitamin A value as butter. Ironically, the form of vitamin A in butter, called retinol, may lack the anti-cancer potential of carotene. In other words, the "natural" butter may lack the anti-cancer ingredient found in "unnatural" margarine.

It is not unusual for manufacturers to add coloring to butter either. The coloring is not mentioned on the label because dairy farmers have managed to exempt many of their products from the rules that other food producers must follow.

Other additives that may have anti-cancer value are vitamins C and E. Vitamin C is often added to food to prevent rancidity and to stabilize the color. We have already looked in detail at its anti-cancer activity.

Vitamin E is used as an additive less frequently. When used, it, too, helps to prevent rancidity.

In theory, vitamin E might help prevent cancer because it is an antioxidant. Some chemicals seem to cause cancer only when oxidized. By preventing oxidation, vitamin E might have value. But research to test this vitamin's value is needed. Don't reach for your supplements yet.

More 100 Percent Natural Additives

The following substances are often used as additives but also occur naturally in the foods listed:

- casein: occurs naturally in milk
- citric acid: occurs naturally in citrus fruits and berries
- glycerin: found in fats
- lactic acid: found in almost all forms of life
- lactose: occurs naturally in milk
- lecithin: found in soybeans and egg yolk
- sorbic acid: found in berries of the mountain ash

Earlier in this chapter I talked of a committee of scientists who reviewed food additive safety for the Food and Drug Administration. These scientists, members of FASEB, concluded that all of the additives mentioned above are safe. The "safe" rating applies not only to the amounts that we currently consume but also to amounts that could be reasonably expected in the future.

The Center for Science in the Public Interest also rates these additives as safe.

The FASEB committee on food additives also concluded that gums commonly added to food are safe at the levels now consumed. These gums also occur naturally—in plants. Food companies use them to thicken and stabilize a wide variety of foods.

You may find gums listed on food labels in any of the following ways:

- guar gum
- locust bean gum, also called carob bean gum

- gum arabic, also called gum acacia
- sterculia gum, also called karaya gum

One form of gum, called gum tragacanth, has caused a few cases of allergy.

Artificial but Safe

Nature gives us her share of unsafe things: poisonous mushrooms, tornadoes, and strychnine, to name a few.

Just as some things are natural but unsafe, so other things are unnatural but safe.

The following food additives do not occur naturally in food. Nonetheless, all are considered safe by both the FASEB additive review panel and the Center for Science in the Public Interest.

- alginate or propylene glycol alginate, used to thicken processed foods
- calcium or sodium propionate, used in breads to prevent mold
- calcium or sodium stearoyl lactate, used in doughs, processed egg whites, and imitation whipped cream
- carboxymethyl cellulose (CMC), a thickener used in beer and common dessert foods
- sodium caseinate, a derivative of milk protein, used in imitation dairy products and some protein-enriched foods
- EDTA (ethylene diamine tetraacidic acid), used in processed foods to prevent contamination from metal machinery
- vanillin, used to give vanilla flavor to artificially flavored foods

The "Uncertain" List

The scientists who reviewed food additive safety for the Food and Drug Administration did express concern about certain additives. They said that a handful of additives appear safe as now used but added that unanswered questions remain. Only more testing, of course, will give the answers.

When other aspects of nutrition such as reducing fat intake are so important, it makes little sense to overemphasize the few additives that fell into this category. But you may want to know which additives were cited. They are

- carrageenan, a common thickening agent derived from seaweed
- several modified food starches
- oxystearins, a modified fat added in tiny amounts to vegetable oils to prevent clouding
- acid-hydrolyzed protein and enzymatically hydrolyzed proteins, used to flavor a variety of processed foods
- several smoke flavorings, used in a variety of foods and spices
- BHA and BHT, two common antioxidants

The FASEB scientists told the Food and Drug Administration that too little research was available to pass judgment on the following additives:

- carnuba wax and Japan wax
- corn silk
- ferric oxide and ferric sodium pyrophosphate
- manganous oxide

- methyl acrylate
- monoglyceride citrate
- sodium ferric EDTA

Strangely enough, scientists believe that BHA and BHT might help prevent cancer. Like vitamins C and E, these are antioxidants, considered to have anti-cancer value by some cancer scientists. No doubt, the pros and cons of BHA and BHT will be much debated during the next few years.

Unsafe as Now Used

Ironically, two of the three additives that the FASEB scientists considered unsafe as presently used were not strange-sounding chemicals. On the contrary, they were household favorites: salt and sugar. Sugar was cited as unsafe for its contribution to tooth decay. Otherwise, though, the scientists considered sugar to be relatively safe at average levels of consumption.

Salt was considered a serious problem for its role in high blood pressure. Tens of millions of Americans have this condition, one of the major risk factors in heart disease and stroke. In terms of the number of people harmed, salt may well be the most dangerous food additive of all.

The third additive cited as hazardous was a little-known one called distarch glycerol. The scientists expressed concern that it might contain traces of a cancer-causing chemical. As a result, food companies have stopped using it.

In short, a decade of debate has made clear that many food additives do appear safe. Some look like troublemakers, and others need better testing. But these are the exception rather than the rule.

Though most additives probably do not cause cancer, it is foolish to assume that none of them do. Each must be studied individually. Insisting that all food additives are safe makes no more sense than saying, "Everything causes cancer!"

11

Naturally Occurring Toxins

We think of nature as a life-giving force, and, of course, it is. But nature has another face. It is responsible for a long list of human woes. Infectious diseases are but one example.

Man-made successes, such as antibiotics and vaccines, have helped us tame some of nature's destructive forces. Scientists are optimistic that we will also conquer the cancer hazards that are part of nature's web.

Among the cancer hazards imposed by nature are some that occur in our food. Within our own country, though, these natural hazards seem to play only a small role in the cancer process.

Possible Hazards in Food

Scientists are hard at work studying the possible hazards in food. Among those that may occur naturally are

- compounds found in food itself
- unwanted contaminants such as mold and chemicals that it creates
- substances resulting when a food is converted to

161

another form—for instance, when milk is changed to yogurt or cheese

Studying the components of common foods is an enormous task. Scientists have only begun what promises to be a long search.

A few of these topics have been studied in some detail. This chapter will tell you what is known about them.

What's in the Coffee Cup?

You have probably noted that the Committee on Diet, Nutrition, and Cancer made no recommendations about the coffee and tea that many Americans drink daily. In its recommendations to the public, the National Cancer Institute also made no comments about these much-loved beverages.

The link between coffee and cancer has been the subject of more than a dozen studies. The results can be described in one word: conflicting. For this reason, neither the Committee on Diet, Nutrition, and Cancer nor the National Cancer Institute has taken a stand on this household staple.

In a nutshell, here is what the Committee on Diet, Nutrition, and Cancer had to say:

- The link between coffee-drinking and bladder cancer does not appear to be a cause-and-effect relationship.
- Three studies have linked coffee-drinking to cancer of the pancreas.
- Some studies link coffee to cancer in other organs, but other studies show no such link.
- Studies on test animals show that roasted coffee

beans may contain a substance with mild ability to inhibit the cancer process.
- Studies on animals also show that something in coffee may enhance the power of cancer-causing chemicals.

Needless to say, it is not easy to draw conclusions from these results.

It is obviously best to emphasize those findings backed by solid research. In other words, it is most important to ensure a good intake of fruits and vegetables rich in vitamins A and C and to limit your fat intake.

I am not convinced, however, that heavy coffee drinking is without risk. My own advice to coffee-lovers is this: keep your coffee-drinking in the range of three to five cups a day (or less).

Incidentally, those who have confirmed heart trouble would do best to avoid coffee. It has been linked to abnormal heart rhythms and to a disorder called VPB (ventricular premature beats). Medical researchers have found that heart attack sufferers who have VPB fare more poorly than patients who do not have this condition.

About the Different Types of Coffee

Cancer researchers cannot say whether instant coffee is preferable to brewed coffee, or vice versa. Scientists also need more time to determine whether decaffeinated coffee poses less (or more) risk than regular coffee.

There has been some concern about the safety of the chemical used to remove the caffeine from coffee. Traces of the chemical can remain in the final product.

In 1975, companies stopped using the chemical TCE (trichloroethylene). Some companies now use a chemical-free process to remove caffeine, while others use a chemical called methylene chloride instead. The safety of this chemical has not been shown to the satisfaction of all. When compared to other aspects of nutrition and cancer, however, this is a very minor issue.

Caffeine, of course, causes "coffee nerves" in some of us. The caffeine content of coffee varies, depending on brewing conditions and the type of coffee used. Here are some estimates of caffeine content per 5-ounce cup:

- regular brewed coffee, percolated: 110 mg
- regular brewed coffee, dripped: 150 mg
- instant coffee: 66 mg
- decaffeinated coffee, brewed: 5 mg
- instant decaffeinated coffee: 2 mg

Memo to Tea-Drinkers

Tea long has been in coffee's shadow. But cancer scientists have been every bit as interested in evaluating its safety.

So far, studies have concentrated on individual components of tea. The best-studied components of tea are caffeine and tannins. Both of these are also found in coffee.

Tannins actually occur in a wide range of plants. Food manufacturers often use small amounts of a tannin called tannic acid. Tannic acid can be added to a variety of products, including butter, candy, gelatins, pudding, and frozen dairy dessert mixes. Breweries and distilleries add tannic acid to beer and other alcoholic beverages.

Caffeine, of course, is found not only in coffee and tea, but also in chocolate and cocoa. Some soft drinks contain added caffeine, though manufacturers are now offering caffeine-free alternatives.

Caffeine: A Close-up

The safety of caffeine has been evaluated by the FASEB. This independent group of scientists reviewed food additive safety for the Food and Drug Administration. Chapter 10 included a detailed discussion of the scientists' study.

The FASEB panel concluded that caffeine should not be "generally recognized as safe," mostly because of its effects on the nervous system. The panel expressed doubt, however, that caffeine poses a cancer hazard.

The Committee on Diet, Nutrition, and Cancer noted that caffeine can cause mutations in bacteria. But the panel found little evidence for judging the ability of caffeine to cause cancer in animals or man.

The Tannins in Tea

The Committee on Diet, Nutrition, and Cancer found "no adequate studies" for evaluating the safety of the tannins we consume. The panel did note that tannins have not shown ability to cause mutations in bacteria. Scientists consider this a hopeful sign that tannins do not cause cancer.

On the other hand, at least one scientist, Dr. Julia Morton of the University of Miami, is concerned about the safety of tannins. She does not insist that we give up tea, but recommends adding milk to it.

Dr. Morton points out that the protein in milk

binds to the tannin. Presumably, this acts like a lock, preventing tannin from having any harmful effects. Whether it does have such effects can only be called an open question.

My general advice about tea is similar to the advice on coffee. Don't overdo it, but pay closest attention to your intake of fat, fiber, and vitamins A and C.

Natural Nitrites and Nitrates

The Committee on Diet, Nutrition, and Cancer advised us to consume "very little" of salt-cured and salt-pickled foods. These foods contain the basic compounds needed for formation of cancer-causing nitrosamines.

Nitrites are the most important building block for nitrosamines. Meat processors, of course, add them to cured meats. These cured meats provide the largest share of nitrite in our diets. Baked goods and cereals also supply nitrite.

Meat processors add not only nitrite to meat but also related substances called *nitrates*. These, too, can pose a problem, but *only if converted to nitrite*. This transformation can take place in the mouth or in the digestive tract. Studies show, however, that only a fraction of the nitrate in saliva is converted to nitrite.

Though nitrates are only sometimes converted to nitrite, it is always possible that foods containing nitrate will end up as nitrosamines. This creates a dilemma. Many foods contain nitrates. The single largest source is vegetables. Fruit juice and water can also provide nitrate.

Yet the Committee on Diet, Nutrition, and Cancer did not tell us to cut back on vegetables or fruit juice. On the contrary, the scientists urged us to eat more of them.

It is another case of weighing the benefits against the risks. *The scientists clearly felt that the good points of fruits and vegetables—their vitamin A and C—far outweigh the potential hazard from the nitrate in these foods.*

The Mushroom Family

The lowly mushroom contains an array of substances with names long enough to make a chemist stammer. As a group, these compounds are known as hydrazines.

Hydrazines have been shown to cause cancer in mice. But, in the words of the Committee on Diet, Nutrition, and Cancer, *"the findings of these studies are not sufficient for conclusions to be drawn concerning the risk to humans."*

Mushroom intake in the United States is not exactly overwhelming. Most of us eat them only occasionally and in small amounts.

At the moment, there are far more important aspects of nutrition to be concerned about.

The Aflatoxin Story

The second type of naturally occurring toxins are unwanted substances that sometimes grow on food. Scientists have long known that bacteria and molds that develop on food can cause infections and allergies.

Only recently, though, did scientists realize that some molds can produce cancer-causing compounds. One such mold produces the well-publicized cancer agents called aflatoxins.

In animals, some aflatoxins show powerful cancer-causing effects. Whether humans are as susceptible as animals is unknown. But impressive studies in

Africa and Southeast Asia have shown a strong link between aflatoxin in food and rates of liver cancer among these peoples.

Liver cancer is not a common form of cancer in the United States. For this reason, scientists have no reason to suspect that aflatoxins are a leading cancer problem here.

The Food and Drug Administration has nonetheless been quite concerned about aflatoxins and limits the amount that can be found in human food and animal feed. FDA officials have concluded, though, that it is impossible to eliminate all aflatoxins from food. This is not a pleasant thought, but it is probably true.

Where Aflatoxins Are Found

The mold that produces aflatoxins prefers to grow on corn, nuts, and cottonseed. Aflatoxins can also find their way into milk, eggs, and meat if the animals were given feed contaminated with the substance.

The Food and Drug Administration believes that its regulations on aflatoxins in animal feed are strict enough to prevent any "measurable" amount of aflatoxins in these animal products.

According to the agency, *vegetable oils made from corn, cottonseed, or peanuts contain no aflatoxins*. It is removed during the processing.

Also, Food and Drug Administration authorities say that *aflatoxins do not occur on fresh sweet corn. Frozen and canned versions of sweet corn should also be free of aflatoxins. The same is true for cornstarch.*

This leaves the following corn, nut, and cottonseed products as potential sources of aflatoxins:

- peanuts, shelled or unshelled
- peanut butter
- other nuts: almonds, pecans, walnuts, pistachios, and so on
- milled corn products such as cornmeal, grits, hominy
- cottonseed or cottonseed meal

The Committee on Diet, Nutrition, and Cancer felt that aflatoxins are mainly a problem in those corn and peanut products that can contain them. According to the committee, other foods known to contain aflatoxins "are of minor significance, either because contamination is infrequent or because only small quantities are consumed."

Aflatoxin Contamination: How Common?

The Food and Drug Administration has tried to find out how often aflatoxins occur in our food. In 1981, the agency tested a variety of corn, nut, and cottonseed products.

Here are the most notable findings:

- Shelled, roasted peanuts were less likely to contain aflatoxins than peanuts still in the shell. However, only a few samples were studied, so these results are tentative.
- Detectable amounts of aflatoxins were found in one of every five samples of peanut butter.
- No aflatoxins were found among seventy-eight samples of pecans. Only 3 percent of walnuts contained aflatoxins.
- Forty percent of milled corn products, such as cornmeal, grits, and hominy, contained some aflatoxins.

Aflatoxins: Some Simple, Practical Advice

The Committee on Diet, Nutrition, and Cancer made no recommendations regarding use of foods that may contain aflatoxins.

Joseph Rodricks, a former Food and Drug Administration official, has offered these sensible suggestions for coping with the aflatoxin problem:

- Discard heavily molded foods or return them to the store where purchased.
- Trim partially molded foods before eating.
- Examine in-shell nuts before eating; throw out those that are molded, badly damaged, or shriveled.
- Do your pets a favor; do not pass moldy foods to them.

Should you avoid peanut butter? Not necessarily. As mentioned earlier, Food and Drug Administration scientists recently detected aflatoxins in only one in every five samples of peanut butter. Add to this the small quantities of this food that most of us eat. We do not eat it in the same amounts that we eat meat or bread.

It is simply impossible to avoid all cancer risks. Also, liver cancer is not nearly as common in the United States as cancers of the lung, breast, and colon.

Therefore, it makes sense to emphasize the foods that help to prevent the major forms of cancer. Doing so leaves room in our diet for moderate use of foods that sometimes contain aflatoxin.

A Look at Fermented Foods

Bread and yogurt may seem to have nothing in common with beer and wine, but they do. In one way or another, all of these foods involve the process called fermentation.

Scientists have long known that a compound called ethyl carbamate can cause cancer in laboratory animals. Yeasts that ferment food produce substances that can react to form tiny amounts of ethyl carbamate.

The Committee on Diet, Nutrition, and Cancer seemed to doubt that the amount of this chemical in fermented foods poses a great threat to our health. Fermented foods provide extremely low levels of this substance—far less than is used to cause cancer in rats, mice, and hamsters.

For this reason, the committee did not advise us to avoid fermented foods. It would be foolish to dwell on such a remote hazard.

It looks as though that old tradition of "a loaf of bread, a jug of wine, and thou" will survive.

12
Cooking Methods

Focus on this chapter if you often eat foods that are high in fat or low in dietary fiber. If you eat few foods of the cabbage family, you should also read this chapter carefully. If your doctor has told you that you have ulcerative colitis or intestinal polyps, you are at higher risk of developing colon cancer. Ask for personalized dietary advice on a regular basis.

Like many scientists, I believe that certain foods can probably help protect us from developing cancer. On the other hand, it seems to me that some foods may actually invite the cancer process.

But new research shows that it is not only what we eat *but how we cook it* that may affect the chances of developing cancer.

It seems that the certain methods of cooking food increase the chances that suspect chemicals will form in it. These chemicals develop during cooking.

Nonetheless, this is not a doomsday story. The facts do not show that all methods of cooking food produce high levels of potentially dangerous substances. *It is simply a matter of knowing the best ways to cook food.*

An Opinion but No Recommendation

The Committee on Diet, Nutrition, and Cancer made no recommendation about the best method for cooking foods.

Dr. Clifford Grobstein, the committee chairman, revealed his own opinion, however, with a remark about broiled meat. "In my family," said Grobstein, "I go unbroiled and my wife goes broiled."

Grobstein explained to reporters that cooking meat at high temperatures—whether over charcoal or in an oven—"clearly increases the mutagens" in it. Mutagens are substances that can damage genes. Scientists believe that most substances that can do so can also cause cancer.

In 1978, Dr. Arthur Upton, who was then director of the National Cancer Institute, revealed this same concern. Appearing on television's "Issues and Answers" show, Upton said: "[In] broiling food we form cancer-producing substances in the process of cooking. It is safer to boil food or to poach food than to charcoal broil it."

Scientists have since learned that cooking meat at high temperatures causes changes in the protein Some of the changed proteins appear to be mutagens. For the most part, the mutagenic proteins seem related to the charring of the meat's surface. Therefore, browning meat in a frying pan probably also causes this problem.

Part Two of the Story

A related problem can result when meat is surrounded by a great deal of smoke. There is at least one cancer agent in smoke that can lodge on the meat. It is called benzo(a)pyrene.

This chemical forms most easily when meat is cooked over, and close to, a very hot source of heat. It also is more likely to form on fatty meats than on lean meats. Charcoal-broiling of fatty meats is the classic example of a cooking method that causes this problem.

Whether browning of foods other than meat results in the formation of benzo(a)pyrene is an open question. It is possible that browning foods such as potatoes also creates this problem. But very few studies have been done on foods other than meat.

How Important Are These Problems?

Not enough is known about these chemicals induced by broiling to say how important (or unimportant) they are. We may hope that protective substances in food, such as vitamin C, might help counteract the effects of these possibly dangerous compounds.

If these mutagens do play a role in cancer, it is probably in colon cancer. If you eat a diet high in fat and low in whole grains and cabbage family foods, you may be at high risk for colon cancer. Why not be cautious and consider other ways of cooking meat? You do not have to give up broiled and fried meats—simply eat less of them.

Even when you broil or fry, you can cut down on the amount of these mutagens by cooking the meat only until the rare or medium stage.

Certainly there is no known harm to baking, roasting, or poaching meats instead—as long as the foods are heated until cooked.

Putting the Findings into Action

The guidelines that grow out of these findings are often easy to follow. Most people, however, will find it impossible to follow the guidelines at all times.

That is okay. You don't have to be obsessed with these suggestions. I offer them simply with the hope that you will follow them when practical. More often than not, adhering to at least some of the guidelines is possible.

Here are the guidelines:

- Favor baking or roasting because with these methods meat is farther from the heat source than with broiling.
- Try to cook meat dishes at lower temperatures by using a slow cooker, simmering in liquid, or roasting in a moderate oven.
- Choose lean meats whenever possible and trim away all visible fat.
- Cook meats in a microwave oven, without the ceramic browning tray.
- Cook meats to the rare or medium stage, rather than until well-done.
- Wrap foods in aluminum foil before broiling.
- Cook foods in a covered container, such as a clay pot, so that no smoke comes in contact with the food.

Making the Most of Meats

As any cook can tell you, some red meats are better suited to these recommendations than others. Here is a review.

For baking and roasting, the best choices are large cuts of beef. These give excellent results when roasted in either a traditional or microwave oven. Round, rump, rib, and tenderloin cuts of beef can be cooked this way. The rib cuts, though, are usually high in fat.

Large cuts of lamb, veal, and pork also roast well. Though the guidelines above suggest cooking meat only to the medium stage, pork always should be cooked until well done. Undercooked pork occasionally contains the organisms that cause the disease known as trichinosis.

Pork chops more than an inch thick can be baked with good results. If the supermarket does not offer thick chops, ask the butcher to slice some for you. You may find them tastier than the thin ones!

Broiling has long been favored for steaks and lamb chops, but you might try baking. You may like it.

More Meat Ideas

Hamburger addicts may not believe me, but ground meat can be baked into some tasty dishes that require no browning.

Meat loaf, of course, is a familiar one. But if you have more than a hour before serving time, you can make easy yet delicious meat casseroles.

Ground lamb, for instance, can be mixed with eggplant cubes and tomato sauce, then baked in a casserole dish. See my layered Lamb Casserole in the recipe section. Ground beef can be mixed with any number of vegetables and baked the same way.

You can even make spaghetti sauce in the oven without browning the meat first. See the Spaghetti and Meat Sauce in the recipe section.

These dishes take longer to cook in the oven than in a frying pan or broiler. Nonetheless, it takes only a few minutes to assemble the ingredients. When this has been done, you need only to let them bake. You can also reduce the cooking time by using a microwave oven.

Cooking meat slowly, in liquid, offers another way to prepare meat without charring it. Cubes of beef round or rump are well suited to stewing. Simmer, don't boil, them. You might also slow-cook them in a crockpot.

The Effortless Beef Stew in the recipe section features beef cubes that are cooked in liquid with no browning.

About Microwaves and Meats

Some cuts of meat can be cooked successfully in microwave ovens. Other cuts, though, sometimes cook unevenly.

The best choices for microwave cooking are meats that are small and uniformly shaped. Lean meats cook better than fatty cuts.

The following cuts of meat can usually be cooked in a microwave oven with good results:

- cubes of red meat
- meat cut into strips of roughly similar size
- boneless roasts
- ground meat
- rib or loin steaks, though rib in particular may be fatty

The beef cuts that are less suited to microwave cooking are sirloin, T-bone, and porterhouse steaks. The latter two are usually high in fat as well.

Chicken without Charring

Every part of the chicken can be baked with good results. You can then use the chicken meat in hundreds of dishes, both hot and cold.

Basting baked chicken with a good barbecue sauce offers a tasty alternative to charcoal-broiling.

Simmering chicken in liquid works best with dark meat. The white meat does not respond as well to moist heat. If you use light and dark meat together, the results will probably be acceptable.

As mentioned in Chapter 8, you can oven-fry chicken instead of frying it in oil. See the recipe for Unfried Chicken for one example.

I suspect that discarding the skin after broiling chicken may be another way around the problem. The mutagens created by charring meat probably occur near the surface. Therefore, the majority of these substances may form on the skin.

My suspicion remains to be tested. But keep in mind that chicken skin packs more fat and calories than the meat itself. For these reasons alone, it is a good idea to eat only the meat.

The versatile chicken can also be cooked in a microwave oven. The results are excellent.

None of the many chicken dishes in the recipe section require broiling or frying. Do try some of them.

Don't Forget Fish

Like chicken, most fish tastes delicious when baked in a moderate oven. Some people disagree, but it may be because they overcook fish.

Most fish takes little time to cook. Fish should be baked only until it flakes easily with a fork.

Just as you can oven-fry chicken, you can also oven-fry fish to avoid frying. Coat the fish with a seasoned mixture of flour or cornflake crumbs. Use your favorite spices and try different combinations.

Again, basting fish with a tangy barbecue sauce allows an alternative to charcoal-broiling.

Steaming and poaching fish are still other options. Fish also cooks beautifully in microwave ovens. I especially enjoy fish that has been baked inside of a clay pot.

All of the fish dishes in the recipe section require no broiling or frying.

A Reminder

When you broil or fry meat, cook it only to the rare or medium stage. This will reduce the level of mutagens. The exception, of course, is pork. It should always be cooked until well done.

13

Will Preventing Heart Disease Cause Higher Cancer Rates?

According to Murphy's Law, "If anything can go wrong, it will." There have been hundreds of more specific versions, covering everything from clothes to computers.

If there were a Murphy's Law of Nutrition, it would probably read something like this: "Change your diet to prevent one disease, and you will get another disease instead."

Apologies to Murphy, but the facts do not support this brand of pessimism. Health experts have long believed that as each disease is conquered, overall life expectancy will improve.

It Happened with Heart Disease

As an example, consider coronary heart disease—public enemy number one. This disease alone accounts for two out of every five deaths in the United States each year. Most victims of this disease have one or more of the following conditions: high blood cholesterol, high blood pressure, or the cigarette habit.

Thanks to efforts to reduce blood pressure, blood cholesterol, and cigarette use, deaths from coronary heart disease have fallen by 20 percent since 1968.

The pessimist would laugh, saying "so people died of other diseases instead—diseases that are even worse than heart disease."

But the statisticians have a different answer. Their numbers show that when heart disease rates went down, overall life expectancy for Americans went up.

This chapter will look at the most important measures of heart health—and how, if at all, these factors affect the chances of getting cancer.

The facts are reassuring!

Cholesterol Levels and Cancer: A False Alarm?

The idea that preventing heart disease will lead to cancer instead comes partly from some recent newspaper headlines. A few years ago, some heart studies showed that men with the lowest blood cholesterol levels had higher than expected rates of cancer. *Not one study, though, found any such link in women.*

These reports led to a massive study of this possibility. The National Institutes of Health contacted dozens of heart researchers worldwide who had collected information on cholesterol levels and health. The scientists were asked to go back to their numbers once more.

The purpose, of course, was to find out if low cholesterol levels were linked to a higher risk of any or all forms of cancer. In 1981, scientists gathered at the National Institutes of Health to take a hard look at the results.

As I waited for the conference to begin, I was a little worried. I had been a supporter of cholesterol-lowering diets for some time. Though I stood ready to change my mind, I was nonetheless concerned that my years of advising people to watch their blood cholesterol levels might have had some unexpected side effects.

Much to my relief, the results did not challenge my beliefs. On the contrary, the findings supported my convictions about reducing fat and cholesterol intake.

A Wrap-up of the Findings

In science, the results of early studies on an issue are not always supported by later research. And so it was in this case.

When the scientists combined their results, they found no consistent link between cholesterol levels and cancer—with one exception. I will tell you about that exception shortly.

Not one of seventeen studies reported at the conference showed any link between cholesterol levels in women and cancer rates.

In men, some studies found lower cholesterol levels among cancer victims. Other studies showed that cancer victims tended to have higher cholesterol levels than healthy people. Nine of seventeen studies showed no link between low cholesterol levels and cancer.

What about those studies that found higher cancer rates among men with low blood cholesterol levels? The scientists talked of the "chicken or egg" question here. Did the low cholesterol level cause the cancer— or did the cancer cause the low cholesterol level?

Some of the scientists proposed that the cancer probably caused the cholesterol levels to fall—something that could have happened years before the cancer was diagnosed.

Important findings by one National Institutes of Health scientist supported this idea. Working with cancer patients, he found that their cholesterol levels fell when the disease was active—and rose when the cancer went into remission. In other words, his research showed that cancer can dramatically affect the blood cholesterol level.

The Vitamin A Connection

More likely than not, the cancer itself has caused the low cholesterol levels found in studies that link the two conditions. But there is another possibility.

Researchers have found a striking link between low cholesterol levels and low levels of vitamin A in the blood. The two seem to go hand in hand.

It is possible, then, that the low cholesterol level is only a sign of what is really wrong: too little vitamin A in the blood.

Whether or not this is the answer, no one can say. But at the conference, one scientist after another expressed doubt that low cholesterol levels cause cancer. I doubt it, too.

The Exception: Colon Cancer

Scientists studying the cancer and cholesterol connection looked first at the total cholesterol rate. This rate combines all forms of the disease.

Their second look considered each different type of cancer. For all forms of cancer except one, at most two of seventeen studies found any link with low cholesterol levels. This is rather convincing evidence that low cholesterol levels are not linked to most forms of cancer.

The exception was colon cancer. Six studies showed a tendency for male colon cancer victims to have low cholesterol levels. By "low," scientists usually meant levels of 180 milligrams per 100 milliliters of blood or less.

Only about 12 percent of middle-aged men in the United States have cholesterol levels this low. Nonetheless, that is no reason to ignore these findings. I think that the research is telling us something.

Explaining the Link

Scientists have long known that some people can eat diets loaded with saturated fat and cholesterol yet keep a low blood cholesterol level. These people are the exception rather than the rule. But they can be found.

Ten years ago, nutritionists like myself used to describe these people as "lucky." But it is time to think again.

People do handle saturated fat and cholesterol that they eat in different ways. Most commonly, these food elements land as cholesterol in the blood.

There are other possibilities, however. Saturated fat and cholesterol can also be changed into bile acids in the digestive tract. These bile acids can then be excreted from the body. We used to think that this was for the best—anything to keep the cholesterol out of the blood. New knowledge, though, requires that we reconsider.

As discussed in the chapter on fats, scientists believe that some of the bile acids encourage colon cancer. These bile acids do not cause the disease directly. Rather, they enhance the power of the substances that do cause it.

So it is no mystery why men who have low blood cholesterol levels could have higher rates of colon cancer. They are handling the fat and cholesterol in their diet in a peculiar way that lowers risk of heart disease but increases the chances of colon cancer.

The Solution Is Simple!

The research here does not tell us that we have to pick one or the other—heart disease or colon cancer. In fact, the risk of both can be lowered by the same diet.

When foods rich in complex carbohydrates (vegetables and grains) replace some of the fat and cholesterol in the diet, the chances of both heart disease and colon cancer should fall.

Health statistics from other countries support this recommendation. In Japan, for instance, the diet of most people is low in fat and rich in complex carbohydrates. The rates of both heart disease and colon cancer are low—much to the envy of health experts here!

A Few Words about Salt

The Japanese diet is not without its flaws. The people of Japan consume enormous quantities of salt. The unfortunate result is rampant high blood pressure. The sodium in salt apparently does the damage.

What about salt and cancer? It is a good question, since the Committee on Diet, Nutrition, and Cancer advises us to "eat little" of salt-cured foods.

Salt has not been linked to cancer. Cancer research points a finger at salt only when it is part of foods that are cured and pickled. Other salted foods have no known role in cancer.

But cut down on salt. We eat much more than we need—about twenty times as much on the average. Though high blood pressure is less common in the United States than in Japan, most researchers believe that high blood pressure would occur even less frequently if we cut back on salt and foods high in sodium.

Salt-Watching Made Simple

There are two basic rules for cutting back on salt: *eat fewer processed foods and go easy with the salt shaker.*

Some of the most common processed foods that are overloaded with sodium or salt are

- processed meats, such as hot dogs, bacon, and luncheon meats
- processed cheeses, such as American cheese and products labeled "cheese food" or "cheese product"; cheeses labeled "natural" *usually* have less salt
- frozen entrées and pizzas
- frozen vegetables that have added sauces; plain frozen vegetables usually have only small amounts of added salt
- salty snack foods such as salted pretzels and potato chips

Most bookstores stock paperback books listing the sodium content of common foods.

Smoking Hurts, Too

Needless to say, smoking does not enhance anyone's health. On the contrary, it increases the risk of both heart disease and cancer.

Cutting back on cigarettes, or better yet, parting with the habit will reduce the risk of both diseases. Much to their pleasure, researchers have found that ex-smokers can definitely benefit from quitting.

It takes time, of course, for the benefits of quitting to take hold. But studies show that as the years go by, ex-smokers gradually attain the lower-risk status of those who have never smoked.

Who could ask for more?

Some Words about Weight

Your weight may affect your chances of developing both cancer and heart disease.

But it is true obesity—not a few extra pounds—that significantly increases one's chances of developing cancer. This is also true for heart disease.

Even when weight does play a role in heart disease, however, it is not as strong an influence as the top three risk factors. These three factors, of course, are high blood cholesterol, high blood pressure, and smoking.

A large study conducted by the American Cancer Society found that seriously overweight men had higher than average rates of colon and rectal cancer.

The same study showed that seriously overweight women had higher rates of cancer of the breast, gall gladder, cervix, uterus, ovary, and endometrium. (The endometrium is the lining of the uterus.)

I hope you have noticed my use of the term "seriously overweight." All too often, people think they weigh too much. From the standpoint of good health, though, many such people are at normal weight.

When people weigh about 30 percent or more above average for their height and age, scientists find a noticeable increase in the chances of getting cancer or heart disease. For those who do not exceed average weight by this much or more, there is often no excess risk of heart disease or cancer.

If Your Weight Is Average

It is hard to make a case for rigorous dieting among people whose weight is just plain average. In fact, the best research I have seen shows that the slimmest among us are not necessarily the healthiest. Recent studies have found that, as a group, people of average weight live longest.

It is important, of course, to understand the perils of serious obesity. But it is also important to be aware that "skinny" is not the only alternative to "fat." There is a middle ground—*normal weight.*

Passing judgment on a person's weight from a book is difficult. Your doctor is the best judge of whether you are overweight. If you weigh fifteen or twenty pounds above "skinny," chances are that you are not obese. On the contrary, you weight is probably normal.

To Sum Up

Scientists do not want to prevent heart disease by causing other diseases instead. They want prevention of heart disease to result in better health.

The factors that help your heart are normal levels of blood pressure, blood cholesterol, and weight. Being a nonsmoker is also a major plus.

None of these four characteristics has been linked to a higher risk of any form of cancer—except colon cancer.

The exception, again, involves men who typically maintain low levels of blood cholesterol (below 180). These men may have higher than average risk for colon cancer. The National Institutes of Health notes, however, that "the magnitude of this risk is generally modest."

In fact, some of the same measures that prevent heart disease seem likely to lessen the chances of some forms of cancer. In summary, research shows that:

- Replacing some saturated fat in the diet with complex carbohydrates can be expected to help prevent *both heart disease and the five forms of cancer linked to high-fat diets.* This is not the case, however, if polyunsaturated fats simply replace saturated fat. All fats are linked to cancers of the breast, ovary, uterus, colon, and prostate.
- Cutting back on cigarettes should lower rates of *both heart disease and some forms of cancer.*
- Avoiding serious obesity lowers the risk of *both heart disease and some forms of cancer.*

Of course, reducing risk is not the same as eliminating a disease. Some people will probably develop cancer instead of heart disease and vice-versa.

Public health specialists look at the overall picture, though. They look at how a measure will affect the population at large. The evidence shows that measures to prevent heart disease should benefit the nation's health—perhaps enormously.

No Retreat from the Dietary Guidelines

Today's advice for preventing disease through nutrition is often called controversial. In my opinion, the degree of controversy has been greatly exaggerated.

As is to be expected, the new dietary guidelines are unpopular with some segments of the food industry. And a handful of scientists protest the guidelines as often and as loudly as they can.

But in my experience, scientists who oppose the dietary recommendations to prevent heart disease and cancer are the exception rather than the rule. No less than twenty international committees worldwide, for instance, have recommended eating less saturated fat and cholesterol to help prevent heart disease.

One of the strongest votes of confidence that I have witnessed dates back to the National Institutes of Health conference on blood cholesterol and cancer.

After several days of presentations about blood cholesterol levels and cancer rates, the conference chairman asked the all-important question: should we change our advice to the public?

The room was almost silent. Only a single scientist rose—to oppose diets rich in polyunsaturated fat. But not one argued that the advice on lowering fat intake should be halted. Nor did anyone protest advising Americans to eat more fruits, vegetables, and grains.

Experiences like this one have convinced me that scientific support for the new dietary guidelines is stronger than ever—and that following them can make us healthier than ever.

14

A Quick
Reference Guide

This chapter contains two charts. The first summarizes the major recommendations in this book. Although I believe that almost everyone stands to benefit from these recommendations, the chart notes conditions that call for special attention to a nutrient or type of food.

The second chart is a guide to food substitutions. These simple changes can bring your diet in line with the recommendations of the cancer experts.

Summary of the Recommendations

Do you?	If yes, focus on:	Try to eat:	Best sources
Smoke cigarettes? Work with hazardous chemicals? Eat pickled or cured foods often?	Vitamin A	Two to three servings a day of fruits and vegetables rich in vitamin A	Yellow, orange, and deep green leafy vegetables
Smoke cigarettes and drink alcohol? Work with hazardous chemicals?	Vitamin C	Two to three servings a day of foods rich in vitamin C, or four or more servings	Citrus fruits and juices and certain vegetables

continued on page 192

Summary of the Recommendations (continued)

Do you?	If yes, focus on:	Try to eat:	Best sources
Eat pickled or cured foods often?		of food with moderate amounts	
Eat large amounts of meat or high-fat foods?	Fiber	Two or more servings per day of high-fiber whole grain foods	Bran and bran cereals, oats, shredded wheat, other whole grain cereals and breads
Eat high-fat, cured, or pickled foods often?	Cabbage family	Two servings per week	Broccoli, brussels sprouts, cauliflower, and cabbage
Eat few fiber-rich foods? Have a family history of breast, ovary, or prostate cancer? Were you or will you be thirty-five or older at first pregnancy?	Lowering fat intake	Limit fat to no more than 30 percent of total calorie intake. Chapter 8 tells you how.	More fruits and vegetables, grains, and low-fat animal products
Smoke cigarettes and drink alcohol?	Lowering alcohol intake	Drink no more than one or two alcoholic beverages per day	"Lite" beers and wines and cordials often have less alcohol than regular beers or wines.

A Guide to Substitutions for Healthier Meals

If you often use:	Substitute:	Purpose:
Beef: rib roast	Rump or round roast Veal roasts	Reduce fat
Beef: porterhouse, T-bone, or club steaks	Round, flank, or lean sirloin steaks; any cut of veal except breast	Reduce fat
Beer	Lite beer	Reduce alcohol
Bread, white	Whole wheat or rye bread; partially whole grain breads	Increase fiber
Butter	Diet margarines or "spreads"	Reduce fat
Cakes, rich or frosted	Angel food cake, gingerbread	Reduce fat
Canned vegetables	Fresh or frozen vegetables cooked briefly in minimum of water	Increase vitamin C
Celery	Carrots	Increase vitamins A and C
Cheeses, hard	Lite-line, Light 'n Lively, or Weight-Watchers reduced-fat cheese	Reduce fat
Cookies	Fig bars, gingersnaps, raisin-fruit biscuits	Reduce fat
Cornflakes, crisped rice, puffed wheat or rice	Shreaded wheat, oatmeal, whole wheat flakes, or bran cereals	Increase fiber
Cream	Milk	Reduce fat
Cream cheese	Reduced-fat cream cheese, neufchatel cheese, or yogurt	Reduce fat

continued on page 194

A Guide to Substitutions for Healthier Meals
(continued)

If you often use:	Substitute:	Purpose:
	cheese (see Chapter 8 for instructions)	
Croutons	Wheat Chex or Bran Chex	Increase fiber
Cucumbers	Tomatoes	Increase vitamins A and C
Flour, white (1 cup)	⅞ cup whole wheat flour, or ½ cup each white and whole wheat flour, or ⅔ cup white flour plus ⅓ cup bran or crushed wheat cereal	Increase fiber
Fried chicken	Oven-fried chicken (see Unfried Chicken in recipe section)	Reduce fat
Half and half	Milk	Reduce fat
Ice cream	Ice milk, frozen yogurt, or sherbet	Reduce fat
Luncheon meats (cured)	Lean roast beef, sliced poultry, tuna salad	Avoid sodium nitrite
Lettuce, iceberg	Romaine or other deep green lettuce, or raw spinach	Increase vitamins A and C
Margarine	Diet margarine or "spreads"	Reduce fat
Mayonnaise	Mayonnaise-type salad dressing (e.g., Miracle Whip) or diet mayonnaise	Reduce fat

A Guide to Substitutions for Healthier Meals
(continued)

If you often use:	Substitute:	Purpose:
Meat appetizers	Fruit salad with berries or citrus fruits	Increase vitamin C and reduce fat
Milk, evaporated	Evaporated skim milk	Reduce fat
Milk, whole	Skim or low-fat milk	Reduce fat
Onion	Green pepper	Increase vitamins A and C
Potato chips and fried snack foods	Pretzels and popcorn (preferably air-popped without fat)	Reduce fat
Potatoes, white	Sweet potatoes	Increase vitamin A
Rice, white	Brown rice	Increase fiber
Ricotta cheese	Cottage cheese, regular or low-fat	Reduce fat
Saltine crackers	Whole wheat or rye crackers; whole wheat matzoh	Increase fiber
Sauces, white or cream	Tomato sauces	Increase vitamin A and reduce fat
Soft drinks	Fruit juice mixed with club soda (see Real Orange Soda in recipe section)	Increase vitamin C
Wine	Lite table wines	Reduce alcohol

15

Cookware for
Cancer Prevention

You probably have decided to make some simple changes in your diet to try to reduce your risk of cancer. You know what foods to stock in your refrigerator and pantry. But what about utensils and cookware?

Certain cooking tools make good nutrition easier—and tastier. *But the last thing that you should do is go out and spend a small fortune refurbishing your kitchen.*

Chances are that you already have the basic kitchenware of a nutrition-minded cook. Some common helpers include

- nonstick pans, pots, and griddles for reducing (or eliminating) fat used in cooking
- a plastic coffee-dripping cone (to make the low-fat cream cheese described in Chapter 8)
- a steaming basket for vegetables

If you do not have one or all of these items, you can find them in most department stores, hardware stores, and kitchenware shops. Needless to say, none will break your budget.

Inexpensive but Especially Useful

In addition to those listed above, the following items will make nutritious food simpler to prepare:

- an egg separator
- a meat loaf pan that drains fat
- a measuring cup or gravy boat that separates the fat from the pan juices
- a salad spinner

If you cannot find these items in a local store, see the "Shopping at Home" section that follows. It lists mail order companies that stock these and other useful kitchen items.

For Serious Cooks

If you spend a good deal of time cooking, you may want to acquire some of the following utensils. Make choices according to your eating habits. If you especially enjoy red meat, for instance, you might want to consider the following items:

- a mechanical meat tenderizer. This is a tool with many sharp "pins" that pierce the surface of meat to tenderize it.
- a meat grinder. It will allow you to make your own ground meat from lean cuts of red meats— or even from poultry.
- clay pots. Lean meat cooked inside of these is remarkably tender—without added fat.

If your passion is vegetables and grains, think about one or more of these kitchen helpers:

- a large steamer that allows you to cook large amounts of several vegetables at once
- a pressure cooker, for quick cooking of vegetables and rice
- a food processor, to make easy work of chopping and grating
- a wok for stir-frying vegetable and grain dishes; only small amounts of oil are needed

Finally, there is one expensive item that also deserves mention: a microwave oven. Some people, myself included, find that vegetables cooked in a microwave taste better than those cooked by traditional methods. Roasts and poultry also fare very well in a microwave. Cooking time, of course, is shorter, too.

Shopping at Home

If you are busy—and who isn't—you might prefer stocking your kitchen by mail. Listed below are some firms that sell useful kitchenware.

Before ordering anything, please get in touch with the companies to confirm that the item you want is still in stock. The prices listed have been taken from 1982 catalogs and may have changed. So again, please get in touch with the company before ordering.

The prices are followed by additional charges for shipping and handling (designated S/H). The charges listed apply if you order that item only. Ordering more than one item will result in a lower shipping charge per item. This is a third reason to consult the firm's catalog before ordering.

Kitchenware by Mail

Supplier	Product
Brookstone Company 5 Vose Farm Road Peterborough, NH 03458	4-cup fat-draining gravy strainer: $17.95 + $3.45 S/H Meat grinder: $24.95 + $3.45 S/H Mechanical meat tenderizer: $31.95 + $4.45 S/H
The Chef's Catalog 725 County Line Road Deerfield, IL 60015	Clay pot, 8-pound capacity: $23.95 + $2.95 S/H Clay casserole dish, 3-quart capacity: $25.50 + $2.95 S/H
Epicure 65 East Southwater Chicago, IL 60672	Mechanical meat tenderizer: $19.00 + $3.60 S/H Salad/vegetable washer: $24.00 + $3.60 S/H 1.5-cup fat-draining gravy strainer: $7.00 4-cup fat-draining soup strainer: $13.00 + $3.60 S/H
Figi's Collection for Cooking Marshfield, WI 54404	Three-tier aluminum steamer: $30.00 + $5.05 S/H Clay pot, 2- to 5-pound capacity: $20.00 + $3.45 S/H Clay pot, 4- to 6-pound capacity $26.00 + $3.45 S/H
Harriet Carter North Wales, PA 19455	Fat-draining ground beef pan for microwave: $5.98 + $2.55 S/H

continued on page 200

Kitchenware by Mail (continued)

Supplier	Product
	Fat-draining hot dog pan for microwave: $7.98 + $2.55 S/H
	Fat-draining meat loaf pan: $6.98 + $2.55 S/H
	Egg separator: $2.98 + $2.55 S/H
Joan Cook P.O. Box 21618 Ft. Lauderdale, FL 33335	8-quart steamer: $28.00 + $3.50 S/H
	1.5-cup fat-draining gravy strainer: $7.00 + $3.50 S/H
	4-cup fat-draining soup strainer: $13.00 + $3.50 S/H
Lillian Vernon 510 South Fulton Avenue Mount Vernon, NY 10550	Salad spinner: $9.98 + $2.10 S/H
	Egg separator: $1.49 + $2.10 S/H
Williams Sonoma P.O. Box 3792 San Francisco, CA 94119	Steel wok, specially designed for electric burners: $28.50 + $3.95 S/H
	1.5-cup fat-draining gravy strainer: $7.00 + $1.95 S/H
	Salad spinner: $12.00 + $2.95 S/H
Taylor Gifts 355 East Conestoga Road P.O. Box 206 Wayne, PA 19087	Fat-draining meat loaf pan: $7.98 + $3.70 S/H

16

Turning Talk into Action:
The Recipes

The following pages are filled with recipes that meet the recommendations of the Committee on Diet, Nutrition, and Cancer. I have designed everything from breakfast pancakes and juices to desserts and snacks—all conforming to my recommendations and those of the Committee on Diet, Cancer, and Nutrition.

The calorie content of each dish follows the recipe. This is the calorie count per serving—not for the entire recipe. If you get more servings from the recipe than listed, the calorie content of each serving will be lower—and vice versa.

A Simple Scoring System

I also have rated each recipe for its content of vitamin A, vitamin C, fiber, total fat, cholesterol, sodium, iron, and sugar. In the case of the two vitamins, fiber, and iron, of course, a high value is good. On the other hand, high levels of fat, cholesterol, and sugar are not good. So "high" can be good or bad—depending on the substance in question.

To get around this problem, I have devised a scoring system that takes a much simpler approach.

My scoring system is easy. Instead of telling you

how many milligrams of this or that each recipe contains, I give a rating of zero to three stars.

***   means *very good*
**   means *good*
*   means *fair*

No star alerts you to a recipe that is a poor source of vitamin A, vitamin C, iron, or fiber—or too high in fat, cholesterol, sodium, or sugar.

For those of you who like numbers, here are the values that the ratings are based on.

The Numbers Behind the Ratings

Nutrient	***	**	*	No Stars
Vitamin A, in IU	1000 or more	500-999	100-499	99 or less
Vitamin C, in milligrams	20 or more	5.0-19.9	1.1-4.9	1.0 or less
Total Fiber, in grams	5.0 or more	3.0-4.9	1.1-2.9	1.0 or less
Total Fat, in grams	0-3.0	3.1-6.0	6.1-9.9	10.0 or more
Cholesterol, in milligrams	less than 25	26-50	51-99	100 or more
Sodium, in milligrams	75 or less	76-150	151-299	300 or more
Iron, in milligrams	2.0 or more	1.1-1.9	0.6-1.0	0.5 or less
Sugar, in grams (sucrose only)	4.9 or less	5.0-8.9	9.0-12.9	13 or more

---

Some Minor Details

You will notice that the nutrient information lists "vitamin A" rather than carotene. Both animal and vegetable forms of vitamin A are credited in the nutrient analysis, despite the possibility that only the vegetable form (carotene) has anti-cancer value.

The reason for this designation is simple. I could not obtain any values for carotene in food. All the food tables combine carotene with animal forms of vitamin A.

The same problem arose for fiber and sugar. For too many foods, values for the insoluble fiber were nowhere to be found. For this reason, I have calculated the total fiber content. It is likely, however, that only insoluble form offers cancer protection.

For sugar, the ratings are based on only one form of sugar: sucrose. Sucrose and table sugar are the same thing. Fruits, however, contain both sucrose and other forms of sugar, glucose and fructose. Good data on the glucose and fructose content of food are scarce. Values for lactose, the type of sugar in milk, are also hard to find.

If the amount of an ingredient is listed as a range, the calorie count and ratings are based on the average amount. For example, if the recipe calls for two to three cups of flour, the nutrient information is based on two and one-half cups.

Finding the Recipe You Want

The recipes are broken into four sections. Within each section, the recipes are arranged as follows:

BREAKFAST FOODS
pancakes
fruit juice

LUNCHEON FOODS
appetizers
main-course salads

vegetable and fruit salads
soups and sandwiches
breads and muffins

DINNER RECIPES
fish entrées
poultry entrées
red meat entrées
main dish casseroles
vegetable and pasta side dishes

SNACKS AND DESSERTS
beverages
desserts

Enough talk. Let's eat!

Breakfast Foods

Sweet Potato Pancakes

1 cup presifted flour	⅔ cup cooked, mashed
1 teaspoon baking	sweet potatoes
powder	1 tablespoon margarine
2 tablespoon sugar	or butter, melted
2 dashes cinnamon	1 egg beaten
1 dash ground cloves	1 to 1¼ cups skim milk

Stir together the flour, baking powder, sugar, and spices in a large bowl. In a separate bowl, combine the remaining ingredients and mix with a fork until smooth and thoroughly blended.

Add the liquid ingredients to the dry and mix with a spatula just until blended.

Spray a griddle with nonstick cooking spray. For each pancake, drop about two tablespoons of batter onto griddle. Cook until undersides are nicely browned. Turn and brown other side.

Serve with maple syrup or applesauce.

Makes about sixteen 4-inch pancakes—about three servings.

Nutrient	Rating	Nutrient	Rating
Calories	280	Vitamin C	**
Total Fat	*	Sodium	*
Cholesterol	*	Iron	**
Total Fiber	*	Sugar	
Vitamin A	***		

Potato Pancakes

3 cups grated potato (2 large)
¼ cup onion, grated
1 egg
⅓ cup low-fat cottage cheese
¼ cup all-purpose flour
¼ teaspoon (or less) salt
black pepper to taste
½ teaspoon baking powder

Blot any excess liquid from the potatoes and onion with a paper towel. (Note: The standard grating blade of some food processors will not grate the potato thin enough for it to cook fully. Use a hand grater for best results.) Stir the potato and onion together in a large bowl.

Process the egg and cottage cheese in a blender until smooth. Add the liquid mixture to the potatoes and onion. Stir in the flour, then add the salt, pepper, and baking powder. Mix thoroughly.

Spray a nonstick griddle with nonstick cooking spray. Heat until warm—not hot. Spoon about two tablespoons of batter onto griddle for each pancake. Flatten with the back of a spatula.

Cook until undersides are brown. For best results,

cover griddle with a lid during cooking. Turn pancakes once and brown the other side. To keep warm until serving, store in a 200° oven.
Serve with applesauce
     Makes ten 3-inch pancakes, about three servings.

Nutrient	Rating	Nutrient	Rating
Calories	220	Vitamin C	***
Total Fat	***	Sodium	*
Cholesterol	*	Iron	**
Total Fiber	*	Sugar	***
Vitamin A	*		

Apple Brancakes

1 6-ounce can frozen apple juice concentrate, thawed to room temperature
1 cup warm water
1 egg

2 tablespoons oil
1⅓ cups all-purpose flour, preferably quick-mixing type
½ teaspoon baking soda
½ teaspoon cinnamon

TOPPING
1 20-ounce can sliced apples, unsweetened
Cinnamon sugar or brown sugar to taste (optional)

     Combine the apple juice concentrate and water. Mixture should be about room temperature. Pour over bran in a medium bowl and allow to sit until bran is softened—about 10 to 20 minutes.
     Beat the egg and oil together in a small bowl. In a separate bowl, stir together the flour, baking soda, and cinnamon. Add the egg and bran mixture to the dry ingredients. Stir until blended.
     Spray a nonstick griddle with nonstick cooking spray. Heat until warm—not hot. For each pancake, drop about two tablespoons of batter onto griddle.

Cook until undersides are nicely browned. Turn and cook other side.

Warm the apple slices in a saucepan. Assemble slices on top of pancakes. Sweeten to taste with cinnamon sugar or brown sugar, if desired. Apple pie filling may be used in place of the sliced apples, but it will be too sweet for some palates.

Makes twenty-four 3-inch pancakes, or about five servings.

Nutrient	Rating	Nutrient	Rating
Calories	344	Vitamin C	**
Total Fat	*	Sodium	*
Cholesterol	*	Iron	***
Total Fiber	***	Sugar	
Vitamin A	**		

Protein-Packed Pancakes

A high-protein, low-fat breakfast that is also rich in iron and other trace minerals.

¾ cup all-purpose flour
¼ cup plus 2 table-
  spoons wheat germ
  with honey
½ teaspoon baking
  powder
½ teaspoon baking soda
1 egg

½ cup low-fat cottage
  cheese
⅓ cup frozen apple juice
  concentrate, thawed
⅔ cup water
1 teaspoon vanilla

Stir together the flour, wheat germ, baking powder, and baking soda. Process the remaining ingredients in a blender until smooth.

Add the liquid mixture to the dry ingredients. Blend with a rubber spatula just until thoroughly mixed.

Spray a nonstick griddle with nonstick cooking spray. Heat until warm—not hot. For each pancake, drop about two tablespoons of batter onto griddle. Cook until undersides are nicely browned. Turn once and brown other side.

Serve warm with syrup, peach sauce, or applesauce. Makes about 16 3-inch pancakes, about three servings.

Nutrient	Rating	Nutrient	Rating
Calories	290	Vitamin C	*
Total Fat	**	Sodium	
Cholesterol	*	Iron	***
Total Fiber	*	Sugar	**
Vitamin A	*		

Orange-Apricot Nectar

3 cups orange juice (fresh or from concentrate)
1 12-ounce can apricot nectar

Combine ingredients in a 1½-quart pitcher. Mix briskly. Chill before serving.

Makes six servings, each ¾ cup.

Nutrient	Rating	Nutrient	Rating
Calories	88	Vitamin C	***
Total Fat	***	Sodium	***
Cholesterol	***	Iron	
Total Fiber		Sugar	**
Vitamin A	**		

Luncheon Foods

Tangy Stuffed Tomatoes

2 large tomatoes, firm and ripe   **2 tablespoons plain low-fat yogurt**

2 tablespoons onion, chopped fine

¼ cup green pepper, chopped fine

½ cup chicken, cooked, skinned, and diced

1 tablespoon mayonnaise-type salad dressing

½ teaspoon seafood seasoning

Slice off tops of tomatoes. Scoop out the pulp with a tablespoon, leaving about ¼ inch of pulp around skin so that a firm shell remains.

Chop the pulp coarse, draining off any excess water. Combine pulp and remaining ingredients in a medium bowl. Stir until mixed.

Spoon mixture back into tomato shells.

Makes two servings.

Nutrient	Rating	Nutrient	Rating
Calories	180	Vitamin C	***
Total Fat	**	Sodium	**
Cholesterol	*	Iron	**
Total Fiber	*	Sugar	***
Vitamin A	***		

Dill-lightful Macaroni Salad

2 medium cucumbers

⅓ cup onion, chopped

¼ teaspoon onion salt

1 cup elbow macaroni, uncooked

½ cup plain low-fat yogurt

½ teaspoon dill weed

¼ teaspoon dry mustard

¼ teaspoon garlic salt

2-3 tablespoons white wine vinegar

Pare the cucumbers and slice in half lengthwise. Scoop out pulp with a teaspoon and discard. Slice cucumber thinly, then slice these pieces in half. Toss cucumber pieces, onion, and onion salt in a large bowl.

Cook the macaroni until tender. Drain in a colander, then rinse with cold water to cool. Process the remaining ingredients in a blender until smooth.

Add cooled macaroni to cucumber mixture. Pour yogurt mixture over these ingredients. Toss to coat evenly.

For a richer taste, add one tablespoon of olive oil. Season to taste with pepper or other spices.

Serve with sliced chicken sandwiches and sliced tomatoes.

Makes four servings.

Nutrient	Rating	Nutrient	Rating
Calories	81	Vitamin C	**
Total Fat	***	Sodium	*
Cholesterol	***	Iron	*
Total Fiber		Sugar	***
Vitamin A			

Orange-Raisin Ham Rolls

1 cup low-fat cottage cheese
4 ounces neufchatel cheese (half of an 8-ounce package)
½ cup frozen orange juice concentrate, thawed
½ cup raisins
12 thin slices lean luncheon ham
2 navel oranges, sectioned

With an electric mixer or blender, whip cottage cheese, neufchatel cheese, and orange juice concentrate until smooth. Stir in raisins.

Place two tablespoons of the mixture in a line, about three-fourths of an inch from the edge of a ham slice. Fold the close edge of the ham over the filling, then roll up and fasten with a toothpick. Repeat this procedure for each slice of ham.

If desired, warm ham slices by wrapping in aluminum foil and heating in a 350° oven for 5 to 8 minutes. Ham rolls may also be served cold.

Arrange the ham rolls on a plate. Garnish with the orange sections.

Makes six servings of two ham rolls each.

Nutrient	Rating	Nutrient	Rating
Calories	250	Vitamin C	***
Total Fat		Sodium	
Cholesterol	**	Iron	**
Total Fiber		Sugar	**
Vitamin A	**		

Luncheon Stuffed Peppers

3 cups cooked elbow macaroni
1 tart apple, diced
3 chicken franks, cooked and sliced
⅓ cup celery, diced fine
⅓ cup onion, chopped
¼ cup plain low-fat yogurt

2 tablespoons mayonnaise-type salad dressing
¼ teaspoon dry mustard
2 dashes cayenne pepper
4 large green peppers
paprika

Combine the macaroni, apple, franks, celery, and onion in a large bowl. In a small bowl, stir together the yogurt, salad dressing, dry mustard, and cayenne pepper.

Cut the green peppers in half width-wise. Remove inner membrane and seeds. Spoon salad mixture into each half. Sprinkle with paprika; chill. At serving time, garnish with any remaining salad mixture.

Makes four servings.

Nutrient	Rating	Nutrient	Rating
Calories	320	Vitamin C	***
Total Fat		Sodium	
Cholesterol	***	Iron	***
Total Fiber	***	Sugar	***
Vitamin A	**		

Tropical Chicken Salad

This recipe was inspired by one in *Thumbs Up*, a publication of Giant Food, Inc.

2 cups chicken, cooked, skinned, and diced
3 tablespoons onion, chopped fine
½ cup green peas, cooked
¼ cup raisins (optional)
3 tablespoons plain low-fat yogurt
2 tablespoons mayonnaise-type salad dressing
½ to 1 teaspoon dry mustard or curry powder
2 papayas

Combine the chicken, onion, peas, and raisins in a large bowl. In a small bowl, stir together the yogurt and salad dressing. Add spices to taste. Add the yogurt mixture to the main ingredients. Stir to coat evenly.

Slice papaya in half lengthwise. Remove seeds. Stuff with chicken salad; refrigerate until serving time.

Makes four servings.

Nutrient	Rating	Nutrient	Rating
Calories	260	Vitamin C	***
Total Fat	**	Sodium	***
Cholesterol	*	Iron	***

Total Fiber   **   Sugar   ***
Vitamin A   ***

Splendid Spinach Salad

6 cups raw spinach, torn   2 tablespoons oil
  into pieces   1½ teaspoons white
2 oranges, sectioned   wine vinegar
8 cherry tomatoes,   few pinches dry
  halved or quartered   mustard
3 tablespoons orange
  juice

Combine the spinach, orange sections, and tomatoes in a large salad bowl. (You may also make
individual servings by combining one and one-half
cups spinach, half an orange, sectioned, and two
cherry tomatoes in a small bowl.)

Put remaining ingredients in a cruet or covered
jar. Shake to blend. Season salad with dressing.

Makes four servings.

Nutrient	Rating	Nutrient	Rating
Calories	140	Vitamin C	***
Total Fat	*	Sodium	***
Cholesterol	***	Iron	***
Total Fiber	***	Sugar	***
Vitamin A	***		

Mexican Tuna

1 6.5-ounce can water-   2 tablespoons mayon-
  packed tuna   naise-type salad
3 tablespoons green   dressing
  chilies, chopped   ¼ teaspoon ground
2 tablespoons onion,   cumin
  chopped fine   1 tomato, sliced

¼ **cup low-fat cottage**   **paprika**
 cheese

Drain the tuna. Combine it with all ingredients except tomato and paprika. Mix until blended.

Spread tuna mixture on bread or crackers. Sprinkle with paprika. Garnish with the sliced tomato.

Makes three servings.

Nutrient	Rating	Nutrient	Rating
Calories	150	Vitamin C	**
Total Fat	**	Sodium	
Cholesterol	**	Iron	*
Total Fiber		Sugar	***
Vitamin A	***		

Bean and Artichoke Salad

1 15-ounce can great   **1 tablespoon onion,**
 northern beans   **grated fine**
1 6-ounce jar marinated   **black pepper to taste**
 artichoke hearts

Place the beans in a colander. Rinse with water and transfer to a medium bowl. Drain the artichokes of as much liquid as possible. Cut into bite-size pieces.

Stir the artichoke pieces and grated onion into the beans. Season to taste with black pepper. This salad tastes best if served immediately.

Makes four servings.

Nutrient	Rating	Nutrient	Rating
Calories	121	Vitamin C	*
Total Fat	*	Sodium	no values available

Cholesterol	***	Iron	**
Total Fiber	***	Sugar	***
Vitamin A			

Creamy Coleslaw

3 cups coarsely
  shredded cabbage
1 cup carrots, grated
  course
1 medium apple, grated
  or diced

½ cup part-skim
  ricotta cheese
½ cup plain yogurt
3 tablespoons apple
  juice concentrate,
  thawed

Combine the cabbage, carrots, and apple in a large bowl. Process the remaining ingredients in a blender until smooth. Pour over main ingredients; toss to coat.

Serve the same day as prepared.

Makes four servings.

Nutrient	Rating	Nutrient	Rating
Calories	130	Vitamin C	***
Total Fat	***	Sodium	*
Cholesterol	***	Iron	*
Total Fiber	**	Sugar	**
Vitamin A	***		

Summer Fruit Salad

1⅓ cups ripe peaches,
  diced
1⅓ cups cherries, halved
  and pitted

2 large bananas
2 8-ounce containers
  vanilla low-fat yogurt

Combine peaches and cherries; chill. Refrigerate bananas. At serving time, slice the bananas and add to other fruit. Top each serving with one-half cup of yogurt.

Makes four servings.

Nutrient	Rating	Nutrient	Rating
Calories	180	Vitamin C	**
Total Fat	***	Sodium	**
Cholesterol	***	Iron	*
Total Fiber	**	Sugar	*
Vitamin A	***		

Crowned Fruit Salad

1 medium cantaloupe	1 cup fresh straw-berries, sliced
2 large bananas, sliced	2 8-ounce containers lemon low-fat yogurt

Cut the cantaloupe into balls or chunks. Toss with bananas and berries. Divide into individual servings. Top each with one-fourth to one-half cup of yogurt. Serve immediately. (If preparing well in advance of serving, toss bananas with some lemon juice to prevent discoloring.)

Makes four servings.

Nutrient	Rating	Nutrient	Rating
Calories	180	Vitamin C	***
Total Fat	***	Sodium	**
Cholesterol	***	Iron	**
Total Fiber	***	Sugar	
Vitamin A	***		

Deliciously Different Tuna Sandwiches

½ cup plain low-fat yogurt	2 tablespoons dates, chopped
1½ tablespoons mayon-naise-type salad dressing	1 tablespoon onion, chopped fine
	3 whole wheat pocket

breads (also called   1 6.5-ounce can water-
  pita bread)   packed tuna
                              ½ cup apple, chopped

Place the yogurt in a paper coffee filter; put into
the plastic dripping cone. Cover with plastic wrap.
Allow to sit over a mug in the refrigerator until one
tablespoon of liquid has filtered out into the mug—
about 60 to 90 minutes.

Combine about two-thirds of the thickened yogurt
with the salad dressing. Combine the tuna, apple,
dates, and onion in a medium bowl. Add yogurt-
salad dressing mixture and blend. If more dressing
is desired, add the remaining yogurt.

Fill pocket breads with this mixture.

Makes three sandwiches.

Nutrient	Rating	Nutrient	Rating
Calories	250	Vitamin C	*
Total Fat	**	Sodium	
Cholesterol	***	Iron	***
Total Fiber	**	Sugar	**
Vitamin A	*		

Ham Sandwich with Vitamin C

1½ tablespoons re-   1 5″-long sandwich roll
  duced-fat cream   (or kaiser roll)
  cheese   2 thin slices boiled ham
1½ tablespoons low-fat   2 slices tomato
  cottage cheese
3 tablespoons green
  pepper, chopped fine

Combine the cream cheese, cottage cheese, and
chopped pepper in a small bowl. Mix until smooth.
Spread on one side of the roll. Cover with ham and
tomato slices. Top with other side of the roll.

Serve with a glass of orange juice.
Makes one serving.

Nutrient	Rating	Nutrient	Rating
Calories	290	Vitamin C	***
Total Fat	*	Sodium	
Cholesterol	**	Iron	***
Total Fiber	*	Sugar	***
Vitamin A	**		

Spiced Cabbage Soup

4 cups cabbage,
shredded coarse
½ cup onion, chopped
4 cups (two 16-ounce
cans) tomato sauce
1 teaspoon instant
chicken soup granules
(or one bouillon cube)
2 cups hot water

⅛ teaspoon garlic,
chopped
1 teaspoon Italian
seasoning
1 bay leaf
1 green pepper,
chopped
black pepper

Combine the cabbage, onion, and tomato sauce in a large pot or dutch oven. Dissolve the soup granules (or bouillon cube) in the water and add to pot. Stir in the garlic, Italian seasoning, and bay leaf. Simmer, covered, for 15 minutes.

Add the chopped pepper to soup. Simmer, uncovered, until pepper and cabbage are tender—about 15 minutes. Remove bay leaf. Season to taste with black pepper, if desired.

Serve with warm bran muffins.
Makes six servings.

Nutrient	Rating	Nutrient	Rating
Calories	81	Vitamin C	***
Total Fat	***	Sodium	
Cholesterol	***	Iron	**

Total Fiber	*	Sugar	***
Vitamin A	***		

My Best Bran Muffins

Even white bread addicts will go for these.

1 cup all-bran cereal	½ teaspoon baking soda
½ cup light brown sugar, lightly packed	1 egg
	¼ cup honey
1¼ cups all-purpose flour	3 tablespoons oil
	1 cup buttermilk
1 teaspoon baking powder	

Preheat oven to 375°. In a large bowl, stir together the bran cereal, brown sugar, flour, baking powder, and baking soda.

In a medium bowl, beat the egg. Add the honey and oil, beating with a fork until smooth. Add the buttermilk and stir to blend.

Stir the liquid ingredients into the flour mixture. Blend with a rubber spatula just until thoroughly mixed. Use a minimum of strokes.

Spray a muffin tin with nonstick cooking spray. Fill with batter. Bake at 375° until golden brown—about 20 minutes. Cool briefly before unmolding. Serve warm.

Makes twelve servings (each one muffin).

Nutrient	Rating	Nutrient	Rating
Calories	150	Vitamin C	*
Total Fat	**	Sodium	**
Cholesterol	***	Iron	**
Total Fiber	*	Sugar	*
Vitamin A	*		

Orange Bran Bread

When I've had my fill of reading and writing, I like to relax by making homemade bread. The marvelous aroma and flavor of this loaf make it one of my all-time favorites.

1 medium orange	2 tablespoons margarine
2 packages active dry	or butter, melted
yeast	1 egg, lightly beaten
½ cup very warm water	⅓ to ½ cup chopped
(105 to 110°)	dates
1 tablespoon sugar	1 cup All-Bran cereal
¼ cup honey	2¼ to 2¾ cups all-pur-
	pose flour

Peel and section the orange. Remove any seeds. Place orange sections and about half of the peel in a blender. Process until peel has been grated into tiny pieces. Pour mixture into measuring cup. There should be three-quarters of a cup. If less, add enough orange juice to make up the difference.

In a large bowl, dissolve the yeast in the warm water. Add the sugar; mix to blend. Add the orange mixture, honey, and melted margarine to the yeast and sugar. Stir to blend. Add egg and blend again.

Stir in the dates and bran cereal. Add the first cup and a half of flour. Mix until blended. Add the remaining flour gradually. Dough will be somewhat sticky.

Turn the dough onto a generously floured surface. Knead for 7 to 10 minutes, working in more flour. Dough is ready when smooth (except for bran pieces) and not too sticky.

Place dough in a large bowl that has been sprayed with nonstick cooking spray. Cover with plastic wrap; let rise in a warm place for about 75 minutes. Dough will not necessarily appear to have doubled. Punch down and shape into a loaf. Place in a 8½″ × 4½″ loaf pan. Cover again with plastic wrap; return to a warm place. Let rise for another 45 minutes.

Preheat oven to 375°. (If dough was allowed to rise in oven, remove it and preheat oven before baking.) Bake at 375° until bread is golden brown and a toothpick inserted in the center comes out clean— about 30 to 40 minutes.

Cool slightly, then unmold. Delicious served warm. Makes one loaf, about ten thick, hearty slices.

Nutrient	Rating	Nutrient	Rating
Calories	240	Vitamin C	*
Total Fat	**	Sodium	**
Cholesterol	***	Iron	***
Total Fiber	**	Sugar	*
Vitamin A	*		

Sweet Potato Scones

1⅓ cups all-purpose flour
1 tablespoon baking powder
2 tablespoons sugar
½ teaspoon cinnamon
⅔ cup sweet potatoes, cooked and mashed

2 tablespoons margarine or butter, melted
¾ cup skim milk
additional flour

Preheat oven to 450°. In a large bowl, stir together the flour, baking powder, sugar, and cinnamon. In a separate bowl, blend the sweet potatoes and melted margarine or butter with a fork. Add the milk and stir until smooth.

Add the liquid ingredients to the dry, mixing with a spatula just until blended. Dough will be sticky and somewhat stiff.

Turn the dough onto a generously floured surface. Turn over in flour. Knead briefly, working in additional flour until dough is no longer sticky.

Spray two sheets of wax paper with nonstick cooking spray. Place dough in between and roll to a thickness of ¼ to ½ inch. Cut dough into rounds with a glass or pastry cutter. Place on a cookie sheet that has been sprayed with nonstick cooking spray.

Bake at 450° until undersides are nicely browned—about 10 to 15 minutes. Serve warm with jam, marmalade, or currant jelly. These scones contain little fat, so a small amount of margarine or butter may be added at the table.

Makes six servings of two scones each.

Nutrient	Rating	Nutrient	Rating
Calories	160	Vitamin C	*
Total Fat	**	Sodium	*
Cholesterol	***	Iron	*
Total Fiber	*	Sugar	**
Vitamin A	***		

Hawaiian Bran Bread

1 8-ounce can crushed pineapple, packed in juice
½ cup plus 2 tablespoons water
1⅔ cups all-purpose flour
2½ teaspoons baking powder

½ teaspoon baking soda
½ cup sugar
1 egg, beaten
3 tablespoons oil
⅓ cup chopped dates

Preheat oven to 350°. In a medium bowl, combine the pineapple, with all of its juice, with the water and bran. Set aside. In a large bowl, stir together the flour, baking powder, baking soda, and sugar.

Add the egg and oil to the pineapple-bran mixture. Add this liquid mixture to the dry ingredients. Stir with a rubber spatula just until thoroughly blended. Use a minimum of strokes. Stir in the dates.

Spray an 8½" × 4½" loaf pan with nonstick cooking spray. Fill with batter. Bake at 350° until bread is golden brown and a toothpick inserted in the center comes out clean—about 45 minutes.

Makes one loaf, about ten slices.

Nutrient	Rating	Nutrient	Rating
Calories	170	Vitamin C	*
Total Fat	**	Sodium	*
Cholesterol	***	Iron	**
Total Fiber	**	Sugar	
Vitamin A	*		

Potato Bisque and Biscuit

Soup

1 large onion, chopped
⅔ cup carrots, sliced
3-4 medium potatoes, diced
1 tablespoon olive oil
1 chicken bouillon cube
1 cup boiling water

1½ tablespoons margarine or butter
1 cup skim milk
1 teaspoon parsley flakes
¼ teaspoon black pepper
½ teaspoon paprika
3 dashes cayenne pepper

In a heavy skillet, sauté the onions, carrots, and potatoes in the olive oil for about 5 minutes. Use low heat. Dissolve the bouillon cube in the boiling water. Add to the skillet. Simmer just until the vegetables are tender—about 20 to 30 minutes.

Transfer the vegetables and broth to a 3-quart pot. Cut the margarine or butter into a few pieces and add to the soup. Stir in the skim milk and seasonings. Adjust spices to taste. Heat through.

For best flavor, prepare at least one hour before serving.

Makes about four servings.

Nutrient	Rating	Nutrient	Rating
Calories	200	Vitamin C	**
Total Fat	*	Sodium	
Cholesterol	***	Iron	**
Total Fiber	**	Sugar	***
Vitamin A	***		

Biscuits

2 tablespoons margarine, at room temperature
¾ cup all-purpose flour
⅔ cup potato (about one large), cooked and mashed

1½ teaspoons baking powder
¼ cup skim milk

Preheat oven to 450°. Allow the margarine to sit at room temperature until very soft.

Work the margarine into the flour with a fork until evenly distributed. Add the potato and baking powder. Work in until ingredients have a uniform texture. Add the milk; mix until blended.

Spray two sheets of wax paper with nonstick cooking spray. Place dough between the two treated sides. Roll out to about ⅓ inch thickness.

Coat the rim of a 3-inch round glass with a small amount of oil. Cut dough into rounds with the glass. Place on a cookie sheet that has been sprayed with non-stick cooking spray. Bake at 450° until tops and undersides are lightly brown. These biscuits do not rise very much. They are crisp on the outside, soft and potato-ey inside.

Serve warm with jam and soup.

Makes about seven biscuits.

Nutrient	Rating	Nutrient	Rating
Calories	92	Vitamin C	*
Total Fat	**	Sodium	**
Cholesterol	***	Iron	
Total Fiber		Sugar	***
Vitamin A	*		

Sweet 'n Spicy Pumpkin Bread

1⅔ cup all-purpose flour
⅓ cup regular wheat germ
1 teaspoon baking powder
1 teaspoon baking soda
1½ teaspoons cinnamon
¾ teaspoon ground ginger
¾ teaspoon ground cloves

⅓ cup margarine or butter, softened
½ cup sugar
½ cup molasses
2 egg whites
1 cup canned pumpkin
1 teaspoon vanilla
¼ cup plus 2 tablespoons water

Preheat oven to 350°. Stir together the flour, wheat germ, baking powder, baking soda, and spices in a medium bowl.

In a large bowl, cream the margarine with the sugar until evenly distributed. Add the molasses and egg whites; blend briefly. Add the pumpkin, vanilla, and water. Beat until ingredients are thoroughly mixed.

Add the dry ingredients to the liquid mixture in two to three parts, stirring with a rubber spatula after each addition. Mix just until thoroughly blended. Use a minimum of strokes.

Spray an 8½" × 4½" loaf pan with nonstick cooking spray. Fill with batter and bake at 350° until a toothpick inserted in the center comes out clean—about 50 to 60 minutes.

Makes one loaf; about ten slices.

Nutrient	Rating	Nutrient	Rating
Calories	230	Vitamin C	
Total Fat	*	Sodium	*
Cholesterol	***	Iron	**
Total Fiber	*	Sugar	
Vitamin A	***		

Cheesey Bran Muffins

¾ cup bran
1 cup buttermilk
¾ cup whole wheat flour
¾ cup all-purpose flour
1 teaspoon baking soda
1 teaspoon baking powder

⅓ cup sugar
2 tablespoons margarine or butter, softened
1 egg
¼ cup water
¾ cup cheddar cheese, grated

Preheat oven to 400°. In a small bowl, stir together the bran and buttermilk; set aside. In another bowl, stir together the flours, baking soda, and baking powder.

Cream the sugar with the margarine in a large bowl. Add the egg and beat until smooth. Add the flour mixture, water, and the bran mixture to the beaten ingredients. Mix with a rubber spatula just until smooth. Stir in the cheese until evenly distributed. Use a minimum of strokes.

Spray a muffin tin with nonstick cooking spray. Fill with batter. Bake at 400° until muffins are golden brown, about 20 minutes.

Makes twelve muffins.

Nutrient	Rating	Nutrient	Rating
Calories	140	Vitamin C	
Total Fat	**	Sodium	*
Cholesterol	**	Iron	**
Total Fiber	*	Sugar	**
Vitamin A	*		

Basic Bran Muffins

1¼ cups bran
1¼ cups all-purpose
  flour
⅓ cup regular wheat
  germ
1 teaspoon baking powder
1 teaspoon cinnamon
½ cup sugar

½ cup warm water
3 tablespoons oil
1 egg
¼ cup molasses
1 teaspoon vanilla
½ cup plain low-fat
  yogurt

Preheat oven to 400°. In a large bowl, stir together the bran, flour, wheat germ, baking powder, and cinnamon.

In a separate bowl, mix the sugar into the water; add the oil. Beat the egg in a small bowl and add the molasses and vanilla to it, blending well. Add the sugar-water mixture to the egg mixture. Stir to blend.

Combine the liquid and dry ingredients, mixing with a rubber spatula just until blended. Stir in the yogurt until blended.

Spray a muffin tin with nonstick cooking spray. Fill with batter. Bake at 400° until golden brown, about 15 to 18 minutes.

Makes twelve large muffins.

Nutrient	Rating	Nutrient	Rating
Calories	160	Vitamin C	
Total Fat	**	Sodium	**
Cholesterol	***	Iron	**

| Total Fiber | * | Sugar | * |
| Vitamin A | | | |

Applesauce Muffins

Tender muffins, with just a hint of sweetness.

1 cup whole wheat flour
1 cup old-fashioned oats, uncooked
1 teaspoon baking powder
1 teaspoon baking soda
1 teaspoon cinnamon

1 cup unsweetened applesauce
3 tablespoons oil
⅓ cup honey
1 egg, lightly beaten

Preheat oven to 350°. In a large bowl, stir together the flour, oats, baking powder, baking soda, and cinnamon.

In a separate bowl, mix together the applesauce, oil, honey, and egg. Combine liquid and dry ingredients with a rubber spatula. Use a minimum of strokes.

Spray a muffin tin with nonstick cooking spray. Spoon batter into tin and bake until golden brown, about 20 minutes.

Variation: Substitute bran for the oats if you want a higher fiber content. The texture will be much coarser, but bran-lovers will be pleased.

Makes twelve muffins.

Nutrient	Rating	Nutrient	Rating
Calories	150	Vitamin C	
Total Fat	**	Sodium	*
Cholesterol	***	Iron	*
Total Fiber	*	Sugar	***
Vitamin A			

Dinner Recipes

Saucy Salmon

1 pound salmon steaks   ½ teaspoon cornstarch
1 6-ounce can Spicy-Hot
  V-8 juice

Bake salmon steaks at 350° until tender.

Heat the vegetable juice in a small saucepan until warm. Remove a few tablespoons of juice to a small bowl and add the cornstarch. Mix to make a smooth paste.

Return paste to saucepan and cook until sauce is thickened. Spoon over salmon.

Serve with rice, a green salad, and pineapple juice. Makes two large servings.

Nutrient	Rating	Nutrient	Rating
Calories	230	Vitamin C	**
Total Fat	*	Sodium	
Cholesterol		Iron	**
Total Fiber		Sugar	***
Vitamin A	**		

Honey of a Fish Fillet

¼ cup honey   ⅛ teaspoon tabasco sauce
¼ cup spicy brown   1½ pounds fish fillets
  mustard
1 tablespoon cider
  vinegar

Combine honey and mustard in a saucepan over low heat, stirring to blend. Add the vinegar and tabasco sauce. Continue cooking over medium heat until mixture comes to a boil and thickens. Stir to break up any lumps.

Bake fish at 350°, basting with the mustard sauce before and during cooking. Cook fish only until it flakes readily with a fork.

Makes four servings.

Nutrient	Rating	Nutrient	Rating
Calories	202	Vitamin C	
Total Fat	***	Sodium	
Cholesterol	*	Iron	***
Total Fiber		Sugar	***
Vitamin A			

Stunning Stir-Fried Chicken

1 large green pepper	2 cups chicken, cooked and skinned
1 medium onion	
2 tablespoons (or less) vegetable oil	½ teaspoon (or less) seasoned salt
20 halves dried apricots (½ cup)	black pepper to taste
	3 cups cooked brown rice

Cut the green pepper into strips. Slice the onion. In a large, heavy skillet, sauté these ingredients in the oil.

Place the apricots in a small saucepan. Cover with a small amount of water. Cook over medium heat until soft and plumped, about 5 minutes.

Drain the apricots and add to the skillet. Stir in the cooked chicken; heat through. Sprinkle with seasoned salt or a small amount of soy sauce; add other spices if desired. Serve over rice.

Makes four servings.

Nutrient	Rating	Nutrient	Rating
Calories	434	Vitamin C	***

Total Fat	*	Sodium	*
Cholesterol		Iron	***
Total Fiber	***	Sugar	***
Vitamin A	***		

Lazy-Day Chicken Casserole

I favor cream of potato soup over other creamed soups because it has less fat.

1 pound raw broccoli	3 tablespoons chicken
2 cups chicken, cooked,	stock, skimmed of fat
skinned, and diced	3 tablespoons skim milk
1 10-ounce can cream of	paprika
potato soup	

Preheat oven to 350°. Steam broccoli until barely tender. Place in the bottom of a 2-quart casserole dish. Cover with the cooked chicken.

In a saucepan, warm the soup. Thin with the stock and milk, stirring until blended. Pour over the chicken and broccoli. Sprinkle with paprika.

Bake at 350° for 20 to 25 minutes. Serve with rice and a fruit salad.

Makes four servings.

Nutrient	Rating	Nutrient	Rating
Calories	214	Vitamin C	***
Total Fat	**	Sodium	
Cholesterol	*	Iron	***
Total Fiber	***	Sugar	***
Vitamin A	***		

Curried Chicken and Rice

A high-fiber version of the Spanish dish, arroz con pollo.

1 cup brown rice,
uncooked

2 tablespoons olive oil

½ cup onion, chopped

1 green pepper,
chopped

½ cup carrots, sliced

½ cup chicken stock

1 to 2 teaspoons curry
powder

1 teaspoon (or less) salt

black pepper to taste

1 16-ounce can tomatoes

1½ cups chicken,
cooked and skinned

Cook rice according to package directions, omitting salt. If possible, replace some or all of the water with chicken stock.

Spread the oil in a heavy skillet. Sauté the onion, green pepper, and carrots until the onions are transparent. Stir the half cup of chicken stock into the skillet. Simmer until the carrots and green pepper are tender. Season with the curry powder, salt, and black pepper.

Drain the tomatoes and dice. Add diced tomatoes, chicken, and cooked rice to the skillet. Mix gently and heat through.

Makes four servings.

Nutrient	Rating	Nutrient	Rating
Calories	380	Vitamin C	***
Total Fat	*	Sodium	
Cholesterol	**	Iron	***
Total Fiber	***	Sugar	***
Vitamin A	***		

High-Fiber Chow Mein

1 tablespoon olive oil

2 cups chicken, cooked,
skinned, and diced

1 16-ounce can chow
mein vegetables

1 16-ounce can pineapple
chunks, juice-packed

1½ teaspoons (or to
taste) soy sauce

1½ to 2 cups spoon-size
shredded wheat

Coat the bottom of a large, heavy skillet with the oil. Add the chicken and canned vegetables; stir-fry briefly. Add the pineapple, with its juice. Cook over low heat just until the pineapple is warm. Season with soy sauce.

To serve, spoon skillet ingredients and juice over the shredded wheat. The liquid from the skillet will soften the cereal to the consistency of rice.

Makes three servings.

Nutrient	Rating	Nutrient	Rating
Calories	470	Vitamin C	**
Total Fat	*	Sodium	
Cholesterol	*	Iron	***
Total Fiber	***	Sugar	
Vitamin A	*		

Ginger Chicken with Apples

For a sweeter sauce, use more apple juice and less water.

½ cup onion, sliced
1 large apple, sliced thin
1 tablespoon oil
¼ cup frozen apple juice concentrate, thawed
½ cup cold water
¼ cup dry white wine
1½ tablespoons quick-mixing flour (e.g., Wondra)
2-3 teaspoons ground ginger
2 cups chicken, cooked, skinned, and diced

In a large, heavy skillet, sauté the onion and apple in the oil, over low heat, until softened. Push to one side.

Add the apple juice, water, wine, flour, and ginger to the skillet and stir, over low heat, until blended into a sauce. Add the chicken and heat until everything is tender.

Adjust seasonings. Thin sauce with additional liquid if desired. Serve over rice.

Makes three servings.

Nutrient	Rating	Nutrient	Rating
Calories	310	Vitamin C	*
Total Fat	*	Sodium	***
Cholesterol	*	Iron	***
Total Fiber	*	Sugar	**
Vitamin A	*		

Unfried Chicken

¾ cup cornflake crumbs
¼ cup unsweetened
  wheat germ
½ teaspoon paprika
½ teaspoon garlic
  powder

½ teaspoon (or less)
  onion salt
6 pieces mixed fryer
  parts
½ cup plain low-fat
  yogurt

Preheat over to 350°.

Combine the cornflake crumbs and spices. Skin chicken and pat dry.

Dip each piece of chicken into the low-fat yogurt, then into the seasoned cornflake crumbs. Turn to coat.

Place coated chicken in a baking pan that has been lined with aluminum foil. Bake until tender, about 50 minutes. Serve with corn and a green salad.

Note: You can vary the flavor of this dish by trying different combinations of spices.

Makes four servings.

Nutrient	Rating	Nutrient	Rating
Calories	267	Vitamin C	*
Total Fat	**	Sodium	*
Cholesterol	*	Iron	***

Total Fiber	*	Sugar	***
Vitamin A	*		

Layered Lamb Casserole

1 medium eggplant
½ cup green pepper, chopped
½ cup onion, chopped
¾ pound lean ground lamb
2 11-ounce cans tomato purée

⅓ cup water
1 teaspoon curry powder
¼-½ teaspoon garlic, chopped
black and cayenne peppers to taste

Pare and dice the eggplant. There should be about three cups; if more, reserve excess for other use. Place the eggplant in the bottom of a 2-quart casserole dish. Cover with the green pepper and onion.

Break the meat into bits and place on top of the onions and pepper. Mix the tomato purée and water in a medium bowl. Add the seasonings. Pour over casserole.

Bake, covered, at 350° until everything is tender— about 75 minutes.

Makes five servings.

Nutrient	*Rating*	*Nutrient*	*Rating*
Calories	222	Vitamin C	***
Total Fat	*	Sodium	***
Cholesterol	*	Iron	***
Total Fiber	**	Sugar	***
Vitamin A	***		

Spaghetti and Meat Sauce

1 beef bouillon cube
1 cup boiling water

1 teaspoon (or to taste) basil

1 29-ounce can tomato sauce

½ cup onion, chopped

½ cup green pepper, chopped (optional)

3 cloves garlic, crushed

½ teaspoon (or to taste) oregano

¾ pound ground round

3 tablespoons quick-cooking tapioca

1 pound spaghetti

Dissolve the bouillon cube in the boiling water. In a 2-quart casserole dish, mix the tomato sauce, broth, onion, green pepper, and seasonings.

Break the meat into bits about the size of an olive. Stir into sauce. Sprinkle one tablespoon of tapioca on the surface of the sauce; stir until blended. Add remaining tapioca, one tablespoon at a time, stirring to blend.

Bake, covered, at 300° for two hours. Stir once every half hour. During the last hour of cooking, prepare spaghetti according to package directions, omitting sauce. When sauce is ready, skim off any fat that has accumulated on the surface.

Top spaghetti with sauce and serve.

Makes six servings.

Nutrient	Rating	Nutrient	Rating
Calories	432	Vitamin C	***
Total Fat	**	Sodium	
Cholesterol	**	Iron	***
Total Fiber	**	Sugar	***
Vitamin A	***		

Effortless Beef Stew

1 beef bouillon cube

1½ cups boiling water

4 medium potatoes

6-8 carrots

8 white boiling onions

1 pound lean beef cubes for stew

½ cup madeira wine

1 bay leaf

¼ cup quick-cooking tapioca

Preheat oven to 300°. Dissolve the bouillon cube in the boiling water. Set aside to cool.

While waiting for broth to cool, quarter the potatoes. Pare the carrots and slice into one-inch chunks. Peel and score the onions. (To score onions, draw an "X" in the base of each one with a sharp knife. The cut need not be deep. This allows flavors to penetrate better.) Trim all visible fat from the meat.

Add the wine to the cooled broth. Place the beef, vegetables, and bay leaf in a dutch oven or 3-quart casserole. Sprinkle with the tapioca. Pour the liquid mixture over all.

Bake, covered, at 300° for one hour. Remove from oven and stir gently. Add more water if stew is thicker than desired. Return to oven and bake another 90 minutes, or until meat and vegetables are tender. Season to taste with salt and pepper.

Makes about five servings.

Nutrient	Rating	Nutrient	Rating
Calories	400	Vitamin C	***
Total Fat		Sodium	*
Cholesterol	*	Iron	***
Total Fiber	***	Sugar	***
Vitamin A	***		

Easy and Elegant Orange Ham

½ cup orange marma-
lade
¼ cup dry sherry wine
1 teaspoon curry powder

4 slices ham, cooked,
about ¼" thick
2 medium oranges

Combine the marmalade, sherry, and curry powder. Spread across the ham slices.

Bake at 350° for 15 minutes. Top with orange slices and return to oven just until oranges are heated through—about 5 to 8 minutes.

Makes four servings.

Nutrient	Rating	Nutrient	Rating
Calories	240	Vitamin C	***
Total Fat	*	Sodium	
Cholesterol	**	Iron	**
Total Fiber	*	Sugar	
Vitamin A	*		

Twice Spiced Pork Chops

4 lean pork chops
¼ cup all-purpose flour
¼ cup yellow corn meal
1 to 1½ teaspoons chili powder
½ teaspoon onion powder

⅛ teaspoon (or less) salt
1½ tablespoons margarine or butter, melted
2 dashes cinnamon
⅛ teaspoon seasoned salt

Preheat oven to 350°. Trim fat from the pork chops. Stir together the flour, corn meal, chili powder, onion powder, salt, and cinnamon.

Brush both sides of the meat with the melted margarine. Dip into flour mixture and coat completely. Sprinkle tops of the meat with seasoned salt.

Bake until meat is tender and thoroughly cooked. (Pork is white when well done.) Cooking time will vary with the thickness of the chops.

Makes four servings.

Nutrient	Rating	Nutrient	Rating
Calories	230	Vitamin C	
Total Fat	*	Sodium	*
Cholesterol	**	Iron	***
Total Fiber		Sugar	***
Vitamin A	*		

Broccoli-Mushroom Masterpiece

½ cup onion, chopped
⅓ pound fresh mush-
rooms, sliced
4 teaspoons olive oil
1 cup skim milk
⅔ cup swiss cheese,
grated

2 eggs
½ cup low-fat cottage
cheese
½ teaspoon onion salt
1 10-ounce package
frozen chopped
broccoli, fully thawed
2 cups whole wheat
croutons

Preheat oven to 350°. Sauté the onions and mushrooms in the olive oil over low heat.

Scald the milk in a saucepan until bubbles start to form at edges. Stir in the grated cheese. Continue cooking over low heat, stirring, until cheese is melted.

Purée the eggs and cottage cheese in a blender until smooth. Add the milk mixture and the onion salt. Blend again.

Press as much water as possible from the broccoli. In a large bowl, toss the broccoli with the mushrooms, onions, and croutons.

Spray a 1½-quart casserole dish with nonstick cooking spray. Fill with the broccoli-crouton mixture. Pour the liquid mixture over all.

Bake at 350° until casserole is set and top has nicely browned—about 45 minutes. Cool for 10 minutes before serving.

Makes five servings.

Nutrient	Rating	Nutrient	Rating
Calories	230	Vitamin C	***
Total Fat		Sodium	
Cholesterol		Iron	***
Total Fiber	**	Sugar	***
Vitamin A	***		

Sweet Potatoes à l'Orange

1 pound sweet potatoes	⅓ cup orange juice
2-3 dashes ground cloves	cinnamon to taste
½ teaspoon orange extract	

Boil the sweet potatoes until tender. Allow to cool until potatoes can be comfortably handled. Pull away potato skins and discard.

Preheat oven to 350°. Mash the potatoes and season with cloves. There should be about two cups of potatoes; if less, reduce orange juice and orange extract proportionately.

Stir the orange extract into the orange juice. Beat mixture into the potatoes with a fork.

Turn potatoes into a 1-quart casserole dish. Sprinkle lightly with cinnamon. Cover and bake 15 minutes.

Makes four servings.

Nutrient	Rating	Nutrient	Rating
Calories	110	Vitamin C	**
Total Fat	***	Sodium	***
Cholesterol	***	Iron	*
Total Fiber	*	Sugar	*
Vitamin A	***		

Orange-Apricot Carrots

This traditional Sabbath dish, known as "tzimmes" in the Jewish faith, is also a tasty and highly nutritious recipe that will even please children who "hate" vegetables.

1½ cups carrots, sliced	¼ cup frozen orange juice concentrate, thawed
¾ cup apricots	cinnamon to taste

Boil or steam the carrots until tender. In a separate saucepan, cover the apricots with three-quarters cup of water. Simmer until tender, about 10 to 15 minutes. Drain both the apricots and the carrots, reserving the liquid from the apricots.

Mix the orange juice concentrate with one tablespoon of the apricot cooking liquid. Toss apricots and carrots with the orange mixture. If sauce is still cool after it is mixed with hot ingredients, warm the dish briefly, over low heat or in a 300° oven.

Sprinkle lightly with cinnamon and serve.

Makes three servings. Recipe may be doubled to serve six.

Nutrient	Rating	Nutrient	Rating
Calories	150	Vitamin C	***
Total Fat	***	Sodium	***
Cholesterol	***	Iron	***
Total Fiber	**	Sugar	**
Vitamin A	***		

Corn 'n Carrot Medley

1½ cups carrots, sliced
1 10-ounce package frozen yellow corn
¼ cup raisins

1½ tablespoons margarine or butter
cinnamon, curry powder, or other spice to taste

In a small saucepan, cover the carrots with water. Cook until tender. In a separate pot, cook the corn according to the package directions. When the corn comes to a boil, add the raisins. Cook until everything is tender, about 3 to 5 minutes.

Combine the carrots, corn, and raisins. Season with the margarine and desired spices.

Makes four servings.

Nutrient	Rating	Nutrient	Rating
Calories	150	Vitamin C	**
Total Fat	**	Sodium	**
Cholesterol	***	Iron	**
Total Fiber	***	Sugar	***
Vitamin A	***		

Simply Sautéed Cabbage

A terrific side dish, especially good with roast pork.

½ head cabbage	1 tablespoon margarine
1 medium apple	or butter
1 medium onion	1 tablespoon olive oil
	¼ cup raisins

Shred the cabbage. There should be three cups. If more, save remainder for other use. Core the apple and slice thin. Slice the onion; cut rings in half.

In a heavy skillet, melt the margarine or butter. Add the olive oil and stir to blend. Add the onion, apple, and raisins, followed by the cabbage.

Sauté over *low heat*, turning ingredients every few minutes. There will be enough fat as long as low heat is used and ingredients are turned frequently. Cook just until everything is tender. Season to taste with pepper and, if desired, a small amount of salt.

Makes four servings.

Nutrient	Rating	Nutrient	Rating
Calories	120	Vitamin C	**
Total Fat	*	Sodium	***
Cholesterol	***	Iron	*
Total Fiber	**	Sugar	***
Vitamin A	*		

Yam and Fruit Fiesta

4 medium sweet	1 tablespoon oil
potatoes	3 tablespoons raisins

1 10-ounce can pine-
apple chunks, juice-
packed
1 large apple

cinnamon or cinnamon
sugar to taste

Bake the potatoes until tender. Drain the pineapple
and slice the apple thin.

In a small, heavy skillet, sauté the apple slices until
soft. Add the pineapple chunks and raisins; heat
through. Season to taste with cinnamon or cinnamon
sugar.

Slice open the potatoes and spoon in the fruit.
Makes four servings.

Nutrient	Rating	Nutrient	Rating
Calories	252	Vitamin C	**
Total Fat	**	Sodium	***
Cholesterol	***	Iron	***
Total Fiber	***	Sugar	
Vitamin A	***		

Pea 'n Potato Skillet

4 small white potatoes
(⅔ pound)
½ cup onion, chopped
2 tablespoons (or less)
olive oil

1 cup cooked chick-peas
½ teaspoon seasoned
salt (or soy sauce to
taste)
⅛ teaspoon black pepper
1½ teaspoons parsley
flakes

Boil the potatoes until tender. Cut into eighths. In
a heavy skillet, sauté the onion in the olive oil. When
onion is about half cooked, add the chick-peas.
Continue to sauté until onion is transparent.

Add the potatoes to the skillet and toss mixture to
blend. Sprinkle with seasoned salt and pepper, followed
by the parsley flakes.

Makes four servings.

Nutrient	Rating	Nutrient	Rating
Calories	180	Vitamin C	**
Total Fat	*	Sodium	**
Cholesterol	***	Iron	**
Total Fiber	***	Sugar	***
Vitamin A			

Creamy Corn Casserole

1 10-ounce package frozen broccoli
1 egg
1 16-ounce can creamed corn
1 cup whole grain crackers, crumbled
2 tablespoons dried sweet pepper flakes
¼ cup onion, grated fine
salt to taste (optional)
1 teaspoon parsley flakes

Steam the broccoli just until tender. Press out excess water with the back of a wooden spoon. Spray a 1½-quart casserole dish with nonstick cooking spray. Place the broccoli in the bottom of the dish.

In a medium bowl, beat the egg. Add the corn, one-half cup of the crushed crackers, pepper flakes, and onion. Mix until blended; salt to taste if desired. Pour this mixture over the broccoli. Top with the remaining crackers and the parsley flakes.

Bake, covered, at 350° for 25 minutes, or until desired brownness is reached.

Makes six servings.

Nutrient	Rating	Nutrient	Rating
Calories	150	Vitamin C	***
Total Fat	**	Sodium	*
Cholesterol	**	Iron	**
Total Fiber	***	Sugar	***
Vitamin A	***		

Zucchini Pancakes

For a change of pace serve these pancakes as a side dish, with poultry or meat.

2 medium zucchini (about 1¼ pounds)	2-3 pinches nutmeg
1 egg	⅛ teaspoon (or to taste) black pepper
⅓ cup low-fat cottage cheese	2 tablespoons skim milk
1 tablespoon oil	½ cup all-purpose flour
½ teaspoon (or less) salt	1 cup applesauce

Pare and grate the zucchini. Blot out excess water with a few sheets of paper towel. Place the zucchini in a large bowl.

Combine the egg, cottage cheese, oil, spices, and milk in a blender. Process until just smooth.

Add liquid mixture to zucchini. Stir in the flour. Mix until blended.

Spray a nonstick griddle with nonstick cooking spray. For each pancake, drop a heaping tablespoon (or slightly more) onto griddle. Cook until undersides are nicely browned. Turn and brown other side.

Serve immediately with applesauce.

Makes twelve 3-inch pancakes; about four servings.

Nutrient	Rating	Nutrient	Rating
Calories	200	Vitamin C	**
Total Fat	**	Sodium	
Cholesterol	*	Iron	**
Total Fiber	**	Sugar	**
Vitamin A	**		

Feast of Noodles

These noodles melt in your mouth. I could eat the whole batch.

2 cups fine egg noodles, uncooked

½ medium onion, chopped

½ cup carrot, grated coarse

2 cups cabbage, shredded

2 tablespoons (or less) margarine or butter

½ tablespoon olive oil (optional)

¼ teaspoon (or less) salt

black pepper to taste

paprika

Cook the noodles according to package directions, omitting salt. In a large, heavy skillet, sauté the onion, carrot, and cabbage in the margarine or butter. Use low heat. Add the olive oil if needed to prevent burning.

Drain the noodles well. Stir into skillet. Season with salt and pepper; sprinkle with paprika.

Makes five servings.

Nutrient	Rating	Nutrient	Rating
Calories	190	Vitamin C	**
Total Fat	*	Sodium	*
Cholesterol	**	Iron	**
Total Fiber	*	Sugar	***
Vitamin A	***		

Broccoli-Apple Stir-Fry

½ cup brown rice, uncooked

1 10-ounce package frozen chopped broccoli

1 medium onion, chopped

2 tablespoons margarine or butter

1 large cooking apple, diced (golden delicious is good)

1 tablespoon (or less) soy sauce

Cook the brown rice according to the package directions, omitting salt. Prepare broccoli as directed.

In a large, heavy skillet, sauté the onion in the margarine or butter until almost tender. Add the apple and continue cooking until the fruit is crisptender.

Drain the broccoli well. Stir the broccoli and cooked rice into the apple-onion mixture. Season with soy sauce.

Makes four servings.

Nutrient	Rating	Nutrient	Rating
Calories	190	Vitamin C	***
Total Fat	**	Sodium	
Cholesterol	***	Iron	**
Total Fiber	***	Sugar	***
Vitamin A	***		

Glazed Brussels Sprouts

1 10-ounce package frozen brussels sprouts	1 teaspoon sugar
	1 cup tomato sauce
1 tablespoon margarine or butter	

Steam the brussels sprouts until tender. In a small, heavy skillet, melt the margarine or butter. Stir in the sugar until blended.

Add the vegetables to the skillet and toss to coat with the glaze. Stir in the tomato sauce and heat through.

Makes three servings.

Nutrient	Rating	Nutrient	Rating
Calories	99	Vitamin C	***
Total Fat	**	Sodium	
Cholesterol	***	Iron	**
Total Fiber	*	Sugar	***
Vitamin A	***		

Snacks and Desserts

Real Orange Soda

¼ cup frozen orange juice
   concentrate, thawed
¾ to 1 cup salt-free club
   soda, chilled

Mix ingredients and serve.
Makes one serving.

Nutrient	Rating	Nutrient	Rating
Calories	110	Vitamin C	***
Total Fat	***	Sodium	***
Cholesterol	***	Iron	*
Total Fiber		Sugar	**
Vitamin A	**		

Cool Coffee Shake

1 cup low-fat vanilla   1 teaspoon instant
   yogurt   coffee
1 overripe banana   2 ice cubes

Purée all ingredients in a blender until smooth.
Makes one serving.

Nutrient	Rating	Nutrient	Rating
Calories	281	Vitamin C	**
Total Fat	**	Sodium	**
Cholesterol	**	Iron	*
Total Fiber	**	Sugar	
Vitamin A	*		

Burgundy Punch

1 cup orange juice
¾ cup red wine

¾ cup salt-free club
   soda
1 small orange, sliced
   (optional)

Mix orange juice, wine, and club soda. Cover tightly and chill. At serving time, garnish with orange slices. Serve over ice.

Makes five servings, each one-half cup.

Nutrient	Rating	Nutrient	Rating
Calories	48	Vitamin C	***
Total Fat	***	Sodium	***
Cholesterol	***	Iron	
Total Fiber		Sugar	***
Vitamin A	*		

Apple-Wine Cooler

½ cup frozen apple
   juice concentrate,
   thawed

¾ cup dry white wine
¾ cup salt-free club
   soda

Combine all ingredients. Cover tightly and chill. Serve over ice, if desired.

Makes four servings, each one-half cup.

Nutrient	Rating	Nutrient	Rating
Calories	92	Vitamin C	
Total Fat	***	Sodium	***
Cholesterol	***	Iron	*
Total Fiber		Sugar	**
Vitamin A			

Champagne Punch

1 cup extra-dry champagne	½ cup salt-free club soda
¾ cup white grape juice	

Combine all ingredients and serve over ice. If storing this punch, cover it tightly.

Makes four servings.

Nutrient	Rating	Nutrient	Rating
Calories	74	Vitamin C	
Total Fat	***	Sodium	***
Cholesterol	***	Iron	
Total Fiber		Sugar	***
Vitamin A			

My Favorite Munch

Warning: It's not easy to keep your hands off this one. (But don't worry—it's very nutritious!)

3½ cups popped popcorn* without salt	2 tablespoons honey
1½ cups Bran Chex cereal	1 cup dried apricots (about 40 medium halves)
2 tablespoons margarine or butter	

Combine the popcorn and Bran Chex. Melt the margarine or butter over low heat. Turn off the heat and blend in the honey.

Spray a nonstick cookie sheet with nonstick cooking spray. Arrange the popcorn-cereal mixture on the tray. Drizzle with the honey-margarine mixture. Bake at 250° for 30 minutes, stirring every 7 to 10 minutes.

Chop the apricots. Toss with the baked mixture in a large bowl. When cool, store covered.

Makes about six cups—six hearty servings.

*Note: Pop the corn in a hot-air popper if available. If not, use a minimum of fat when preparing the popcorn.

Nutrient	Rating	Nutrient	Rating
Calories	180	Vitamin C	**
Total Fat	**	Sodium	**
Cholesterol	***	Iron	***
Total Fiber	**	Sugar	***
Vitamin A	***		

A+ Apricot Bars

Outrageously delicious!

1 cup dried apricots
¾ cup boiling water
2 tablespoons frozen orange juice concentrate, thawed
1-3 tablespoons sugar
1 cup all-purpose flour
1 cup quick oats, uncooked

⅓ cup brown sugar
⅓ cup sugar
½ teaspoon baking soda
½ teaspoon cinnamon
1 teaspoon vanilla
½ cup margarine or butter, melted

Preheat oven to 350°. Cut each apricot half into three to four strips. Place in a small saucepan and cover with the boiling water.

Simmer, covered, for about 15 minutes—until water is absorbed and apricots have the consistency of a paste. Check the apricots every 5 minutes during cooking to make sure that there is enough water to prevent burning. If there is too much water after 15 minutes of cooking, remove lid and simmer a few minutes longer. Stir in the orange juice concentrate. Add the one to three tablespoons of sugar to taste.

In a large bowl, stir together the flour, oats, remaining sugars, baking soda, and cinnamon. Add the vanilla to the margarine. Work the margarine mixture into the dry ingredients until evenly distributed. The mixture will be like crumbs.

Spray a 9-inch square pan with nonstick cooking spray. Lightly press about two-thirds of the crumb mixture into pan. (Do not pack tightly; lightly packed dough is more tender.) Spread the apricot filling over the crumbs, leaving a half-inch border between filling and the pan. Top with remaining crumbs.

Bake at 350° until top is slightly browned—about 20 to 25 minutes.

Makes nine bars, each 3 inches square.

Nutrient	Rating	Nutrient	Rating
Calories	280	Vitamin C	**
Total Fat		Sodium	
Cholesterol	***	Iron	**
Total Fiber	*	Sugar	
Vitamin A	***		

Luscious Banana Cake

1¼ cup all purpose flour, preferably quick-mixing type
¼ cup plus 2 tablespoons wheat germ toasted with honey
⅔ cup sugar
1 teaspoon baking powder
½ teaspoon baking soda

1 egg
2 medium *overripe* bananas (1 cup mashed)
½ cup buttermilk
3 tablespoons oil
1 ripe banana

Preheat oven to 350°. In a large bowl, stir together the flour, one-quarter cup of wheat germ, sugar, baking powder, and baking soda.

Combine the egg, two overripe bananas, buttermilk, and oil in a blender. Process just until smooth. Pour into the dry ingredients and mix just until thoroughly blended. Use a minimum of strokes.

Reserve three-quarters of a cup of the batter. Slice the remaining banana very thin. Spray a 9-inch square pan with nonstick cooking spray. Fill with all the batter, except the reserved three-quarters cup.

Line the top of the batter with the banana slices. Cover with the reserved batter. Sprinkle the last two tablespoons of wheat germ over all.

Bake at 350° until cake is golden brown and a toothpick inserted in the center comes out dry—about 30 to 35 minutes. Cool slightly before unmolding.

Makes nine servings, each 3 inches square.

Note: Recipe can be doubled. Bake in a 9″ × 13″ pan. Cooking time will increase by about 10 minutes.

Nutrient	Rating	Nutrient	Rating
Calories	180	Vitamin C	
Total Fat	**	Sodium	**
Cholesterol	**	Iron	**
Total Fiber	*	Sugar	
Vitamin A	*		

Strawberry Shortcake

1½ cups all-purpose flour	2 tablespoons margarine or butter, melted
1 teaspoon baking powder	¾ cup plus 2 tablespoons buttermilk
½ teaspoon baking soda	1 teaspoon vanilla

¾ cup sugar
1 egg

2 pints fresh straw-
berries
1 pint vanilla low-fat
yogurt

Preheat oven to 350°. Stir together the flour, baking powder, baking soda, and sugar in a large bowl. In a separate bowl, beat the egg. Add the melted margarine, buttermilk, and vanilla to the beaten egg.

Stir the liquid ingredients into the flour mixture. Blend with a spatula using a minimum of strokes. Spray a 9-inch square pan with nonstick cooking spray. Fill with batter. Bake at 350° until a toothpick inserted in the center comes out clean: about 35 to 40 minutes. When cool, cut into eight pieces.

Halve the strawberries. Your may want to dust them lightly with sugar, depending on their sweetness. Top each serving of cake with one-half cup of berries and one-quarter cup of yogurt.

Makes eight servings.

Nutrient	Rating	Nutrient	Rating
Calories	250	Vitamin C	***
Total Fat	**	Sodium	*
Cholesterol	**	Iron	**
Total Fiber	*	Sugar	
Vitamin A	*		

Razzle-Dazzle Angel Cake

1 10-ounce box frozen
raspberries, thawed

1¼ cups plain low-fat
yogurt
6 slices angel food cake

Drain the raspberries, collecting the syrup in a measuring cup. There should be about one-half cup of syrup. If less, reduce the amount of yogurt proportionately. Combine the syrup with the yogurt. Mix until blended.

Spoon about three tablespoons of the sweetened yogurt over each slice of cake. Garnish with raspberries and serve.

Variation: Add some sliced bananas to each serving. Makes six servings.

Nutrient	Rating	Nutrient	Rating
Calories	170	Vitamin C	**
Total Fat	***	Sodium	**
Cholesterol	***	Iron	*
Total Fiber	**	Sugar	
Vitamin A			

Peach Dessert for Three

1 16-ounce can sliced peaches, juice-packed
¾ cup quick oats, uncooked
2 tablespoons light brown sugar, packed
½ teaspoon cinnamon
2 tablespoons (or less) margarine or butter, melted

Preheat oven to 350°. Drain the peaches. Stir together the oats, brown sugar, and cinnamon. Add the melted margarine or butter. Mix until blended.

Spray a 1-quart casserole dish with nonstick cooking spray. Place about half of the peaches in the bottom. Cover with half of the oat mixture. Add remaining peaches and top with the rest of the oats.

Cover and bake at 350° until tender, about 35 to 40 minutes. Serve warm.

Makes three servings.

Nutrient	Rating	Nutrient	Rating
Calories	259	Vitamin C	*
Total Fat	*	Sodium	**

Cholesterol	***	Iron	**
Total Fiber	**	Sugar	
Vitamin A	**		

Sugar and Spice Cake

This cake takes less time than many packaged mixes.
Clean-up is a breeze, too.

¾ cup whole wheat flour	½ teaspoon ground cloves
¾ cup all-purpose flour	¼ teaspoon ground ginger
½ teaspoon baking powder	¼ cup vegetable oil
¾ teaspoon baking soda	1 tablespoon lemon juice
1 cup brown sugar, packed	1 cup water
1 teaspoon cinnamon	½ cup raisins
1 teaspoon allspice	

Preheat oven to 350°. In a large bowl, stir together
the flours, baking powder, baking soda, brown sugar,
and spices.

Add the vegetable oil, lemon juice, and water. Mix
with a rubber spatula just until blended. Use a
minimum of strokes. Stir in the raisins.

Spray a 9-inch square pan with nonstick cooking
spray. Fill with batter. Bake at 350° until a toothpick
inserted in the center comes out clean—about 30
minutes.

Delicious served warm with a scoop of high-quality
vanilla ice milk.

Makes eight servings.

| *Nutrient* | *Rating* | *Nutrient* | *Rating* |
| Calories | 260 | Vitamin C | |

Total Fat	*	Sodium	**
Cholesterol	***	Iron	**
Total Fiber	*	Sugar	
Vitamin A			

Baked Apples

2 baking apples	**½ cup dry white wine**
1 to 2 tablespoons currant jelly	

Preheat oven to 375°.

Core the apples to ½ inch from the bottom. Peel a strip about ¾ inch thick from the top of the apples. Fill the cavity of each apple with one-half to one tablespoon of the jelly, depending on the size of fruit and the degree of sweetness desired.

Place the apples in a baking pan. Pour wine in the bottom of the dish. Bake the apples at 375° until tender (not mushy), basting frequently. When apples are done, baste again with the pan juices.

Makes two servings.

Nutrient	*Rating*	*Nutrient*	*Rating*
Calories	160	Vitamin C	*
Total Fat	***	Sodium	***
Cholesterol	***	Iron	*
Total Fiber	**	Sugar	***
Vitamin A	*		

Old-Fashioned Oat Crust

1½ cups quick oats, uncooked	**1 teaspoon cinnamon**
¼ cup sugar	**¼ cup margarine or butter, melted**

In a medium bowl, stir together the oats, sugar, and cinnamon. Add the melted margarine and mix until oats are thoroughly coated.

Press mixture into the bottom of an 8- or 9-inch pie plate. (If available, use another pie plate of same size to press into shape.)

Chill for at least 30 minutes before filling. If you are using a nonbake filling, bake the oat crust at 300° for 15 to 20 minutes before filling.

Makes one pie shell—enough crust for eight servings of pie.

Nutrient	Rating	Nutrient	Rating
Calories	140	Vitamin C	
Total Fat	*	Sodium	***
Cholesterol	***	Iron	*
Total Fiber	*	Sugar	**
Vitamin A	*		

Appendix
Further Reading

General Nutrition

Brody, Jane. *Jane Brody's Nutrition Book*. New York: W. W. Norton. 1981. Available in bookstores.

Senate Select Committee on Nutrition and Human Needs. *Dietary Goals for the United States*. Washington: Government Printing Office, 1977. Available by mail. Send check for $2.30, payable to Superintendent of Documents, to Government Printing Office, Washington, DC 20402. Request stock number 052-070-04376-8.

Fats and Cholesterol

Carper, Jean. *The All-in-One Lowfat Gram Counter*. New York: Bantam Books, 1980. Available in bookstores.

Hausman, Patricia. *Jack Sprat's Legacy: The Science and Politics of Fat and Cholesterol*. New York: Richard Marek Publishers, 1981. Available by mail. Send check for $6.95 to CSPI Reports, 1755 "S" Street N.W., Washington, DC 20009.

Fiber

Anderson, J. W. *Diabetes: A Practical New Guide to Healthy Living*. New York: Arco Publishers, 1981. Available in bookstores.

Anderson, J. W. *User's Guide to HCF (High Carbo-hydrate and Fiber) Diets.* Lexington, KY: HCF Diabetes Research Foundation, 1980. Available by mail. Send check for $4 payable to HCF Research Foundation, 1872 Blairmore Road, Lexington, KY 40502.

Burkitt, Denis. *Eat Right—To Stay Healthy and Enjoy Life More.* New York: Arco Publishers, 1979. Available in bookstores.

Alcohol

Center for Science in the Public Interest. *Chemical Additives in Booze.* 1982. Available by mail. Send check for $4.95 to CSPI Reports, 1755 "S" Street N.W., Washington, DC 20009.

Food Additives

Jacobson, Michael. *Eater's Digest: The Consumer's Factbook of Food Additives.* Garden City, N.Y.: Doubleday-Anchor Books. Available in bookstores or by mail. For mail order, send check for $2.50 to CSPI Reports, 1755 "S" Street N.W., Washington, DC 20009.

Center for Science in the Public Interest. *Chemical Cuisine* poster. 1978. Available by mail. Send $3 for standard poster, $6 for laminated poster, to CSPI Reports, 1755 "S" Street N.W., Washington, DC 20009.

Federation of American Societies for Experimental Biology. Summary Table of Final Report, Evaluation of GRAS (Generally Recognized As Safe) Monographs. This table shows the results of a recent scientific study of food additive safety. Available from the Food and Drug Administration, GRAS Review Branch, Washington, DC 20204.

Index

Improve Your Health
with WARNER BOOKS

___**LOW SALT SECRETS FOR YOUR DIET**   *(L37-223, $3.95, U.S.A.)*
    by Dr. William J. Vaughan   *(L37-358, $4.50, Canada)*

Not just for people who must restrict salt intake, but for everyone! Forty to sixty million Americans have high blood pressure, and nearly one million Americans die of heart disease every year. Hypertension, often called the silent killer, can be controlled by restricting your intake of salt. This handy pocket-size guide can tell you at a glance how much salt is hidden in more than 2,600 brand-name and natural foods.

___**EARL MINDELL'S VITAMIN BIBLE**   *(L30-626, $3.95, U.S.A.)*
    by Earl Mindell   *(L32-002, $4.95, Canada)*

Earl Mindell, a certified nutritionist and practicing pharmacist for over fifteen years, heads his own national company specializing in vitamins. His VITA-MIN BIBLE is the most comprehensive and complete book about vitamins and nutrient supplements ever written. This important book reveals how vitamin needs vary for each of us and how to determine yours; how to substitute natural substances for tranquilizers, sleeping pills, and other drugs; how the right vitamins can help your heart, retard aging, and improve your sex life.

___**SUGAR BLUES**
    by William Dufty   *(L30-512, $3.95)*

Like opium, morphine, and heroin, sugar is an addictive drug, yet Americans consume it daily in every thing from cigarettes to bread. If you are over-weight, or suffer from migrane, hypoglycemia or acne, the plague of the Sugar Blues has hit you. In fact, by accepted diagnostic standards, *our entire society is pre-diabetic. Sugar Blues* shows you how to live better without it and includes the recipes for delicious dishes—all sugar free!

___**THE CORNER DRUGSTORE**   large format paperback:
    by Max Leber   *(L97-989, $6.95, U.S.A.)*
         (L37-278, $8.50, Canada)

In simple, down-to-earth language, THE CORNER DRUGSTORE provides complete coverage of the over-the-counter products and services available at your local pharmacy. Here's everything you should know about every-thing that pharmacies sell, a working knowledge that will save you money and enable you to use nonprescription drugs and health aids more wisely.

WARNER BOOKS
P.O. Box 690
New York, N.Y. 10019

Please send me the books I have checked. I enclose a check or money order (not cash), plus 50¢ per order and 50¢ per copy to cover postage and handling.*
(Allow 4 weeks for delivery.)

_____ Please send me your free mail order catalog. (If ordering only the catalog, include a large self-addressed, stamped envelope.)

Name _____

Address _____

City _____

State _____ Zip _____

*N.Y. State and California residents add applicable sales tax.   80

FOR YOUR HEALTH
FROM WARNER BOOKS

___**DIABETES: A PRACTICAL NEW GUIDE**   (L32-946, $3.95)
TO HEALTHY LIVING
James W. Anderson, M.D.

Take charge of your life with the doctor's revolutionary new treatment. Here
is the prescription for a longer, happier, healthier life for all diabetics, based
on a proven–effective diet, discipline and exercise program that finally puts
you in control. Dr. James W. Anderson tells you everything you need to
know.

___**CONFESSIONS OF A MEDICAL HERETIC**   (L30-627, $3.95)
Robert S. Mendelsohn, M.D.

An important book by a distinguished physician who is convinced that
annual physical examinations are a health risk . . . hospitals are dangerous
places for the sick . . . most operations do little good and many do harm . . .
medical testing laboratories are scandalously inaccurate . . . many drugs
cause more problems than they cure. The author provides all the information you need to start making your own decisions regarding your medical
treatment.

___**THE HARVARD MEDICAL SCHOOL**   (L30-104, $3.95)
HEALTH LETTER BOOK
*edited by G. Timothy Johnson, M.D.
and Stephen E. Goldfinger, M.D.*

This book is a clear look at the "latest findings"—sifting, evaluating, organiz-
ing, and translating them into language everyone can understand. In short,
this book helps you separate medical fact from medical fiction.

___**WHERE DID EVERYBODY GO?**   (J30-375, $2.95)
Paul Molloy

Paul Molloy, nationally syndicated columnist with the *Chicago Sun-Times,*
thought he was a social drinker until he was forced to face the truth. In this
candid book, he tells of his struggle and of the discoveries he has made
about the nature of alcoholics, alcoholism, and its effects on families and
friends.

WARNER BOOKS
P.O. Box 690
New York, N.Y. 10019

Please send me the books I have checked. I enclose a check or
money order (not cash), plus 50¢ per order and 50¢ per copy to cover
postage and handling.* (Allow 4 weeks for delivery.)

_____ Please send me your free mail order catalog. (If ordering
           only the catalog, include a large self-addressed, stamped
           envelope.)

Name _____

Address _____

City _____

State _____ Zip _____

*N.Y. State and California residents add applicable sales tax.   75